TRAUMA

Biomedical Library

Queen's University Belfast

Tel: 028 9097 2710

E-mail: biomed.info@qub.ac.uk

For due dates and renewals:

QUB borrowers see 'MY ACCOUNT' at

http://library.qub.ac.uk/qcat

or go to the Library Home Page

HPSS borrowers see 'MY ACCOUNT' at

www.honni.qub.ac.uk/qcat

This book must be returned not later than its due
date, but is subject to recall if in demand

Fines are imposed on overdue books

The KEY TOPICS Series

Advisors:

T.M. Craft *Department of Anaesthesia and Intensive Care, Royal United Hospital, Bath, UK*
C.S. Garrard *Intensive Therapy Unit, John Radcliffe Hospital, Oxford, UK*
P.M. Upton *Department of Anaesthetics, Treliske Hospital, Truro, UK*

Anaesthesia, Second Edition

Obstetrics and Gynaecology

Accident and Emergency Medicine

Paediatrics

Orthopaedic Surgery

Otolaryngology and Head and Neck Surgery

Ophthalmology

Psychiatry

General Surgery

Renal Medicine

Trauma

Chronic Pain

Forthcoming titles include:

Oral and Maxillofacial Surgery

Oncology

Cardiovascular Medicine

Obstetrics and Gynaecology, Second Edition

Molecular Biology and Genetics

Neonatology

Critical Care

Orthopaedic Trauma Surgery

KEY TOPICS IN

TRAUMA

I. GREAVES
MRCP(UK) DTM&H Dip IMC.RCSEd
Specialist Registrar in Accident and Emergency Medicine,
The General Infirmary at Leeds, UK

K. PORTER
FRCS DiplMC.RCSEd
Consultant Trauma and Orthopaedic Surgeon,
University Hospital, Birmingham, UK

D. BURKE
FRCS(Ed) FRCS(A&E)Ed
Senior Registrar in Accident and Emergency Medicine,
The Childrens' Hospital, Birmingham, UK

βIOS
SCIENTIFIC
PUBLISHERS

297482

© BIOS Scientific Publishers Limited, 1997

First published 1997

A CIP catalogue record for this book is available from the British Library.

ISBN 1 85996 175 4

BIOS Scientific Publishers Ltd
9 Newtec Place, Magdalen Road, Oxford OX4 1RE, UK
Tel. +44 (0)1865 726286. Fax. +44 (0)1865 246823
World Wide Web home page: http://www.Bookshop.co.uk/BIOS/

DISTRIBUTORS

Australia and New Zealand
   Blackwell Science Asia
   54 University Street
   Carlton, South Victoria 3053

India
   Viva Books Private Limited
   4325/3 Ansari Road, Daryaganj
   New Delhi 110002

Singapore and South East Asia
   Toppan Company (S) PTE Ltd
   38 Liu Fang Road, Jurong
   Singapore 2262

USA and Canada
   BIOS Scientific Publishers
   PO Box 605, Herndon
   VA 20172-0605

Important Note from the Publisher
The information contained within this book was obtained by BIOS Scientific Publishers Ltd from sources believed by us to be reliable. However, while every effort has been made to ensure its accuracy, no responsibility for loss or injury whatsoever occasioned to any person acting or refraining from action as a result of information contained herein can be accepted by the authors or publishers.

The reader should remember that medicine is a constantly evolving science and while the authors and publishers have ensured that all dosages, applications and practices are based on current indications, there may be specific practices which differ between communities. You should always follow the guidelines laid down by the manufacturers of specific products and the relevant authorities in the country in which you are practising.

Typeset by Chandos Electronic Publishing, Stanton Harcourt, UK.
Printed by Biddles Ltd, Guildford, UK.

CONTENTS

[a]Contributed by J.M. Elliot (MB, BS, FRCA DipIMC.RCSEd), Consultant Anaethetist, Good Hope Hospital NHS Trust, Sutton Coldfield, UK.
[b]Contributed by M. Green (FRCS), Higher Surgical Trainee, West Midlands Orthopaedic Training Rotation, West Midlands, UK.
[c]Contributed by S. Bradley (MB, ChB, FRCR), Consultant Radiologist, University Hospital, Birmingham, UK.
[d]Contributed by A. Gray (FRCS(A&E)Ed), Research Fellow in Accident and Emergency Medicine, St James's University Hospital, Leeds, UK.
[e]Contributed by P.V. Dyer (FFDRCSI, FRCS(Ed)), Senior Registrar in Maxillofacial Surgery, Royal London Hospital, London, UK.
[f]Contributed by D.A. Alexander (FRC Psych), Professor of Mental Health, University of Aberdeen, Aberdeen, UK.

ABBREVIATIONS

A&E	accident and emergency
ADH	antidiuretic hormone
AIS	abbreviated injury scale
AP	anterio-posterior
ARC	AIDS-related complex
ARDS	adult respiratory distress syndrome
ARF	acute renal failure
ATFL	anterior talofibular ligament
ATLS	Advanced Trauma Life Support
ATNC	Advance Trauma Nursing Certificate
AV	arterio-venous
AXR	abdominal X-ray
BNF	British National Formulary
BP	blood pressure
BSA	body surface area
CAA	Civil Aviation Authority
CFL	calcaneofibular ligament
CFS	cerebrospinal injury
CPR	cardiopulmonary resuscitation
CT	computed tomography
CVP	central venous pressure
CXR	chest X-ray
DIC	disseminated intravascular coagulation
DIPJ	distal interphalangeal joint
DPL	diagnostic peritoneal lavage
DVT	deep vein thrombosis
ECG	electrocardiogram
ECMO	extracorporeal membrane oxygenation
EMD	electro mechanical dissociation
$ETCO_2$	end-tidal carbon dioxide concentration
FDP	flexor digitorum profundus
FDS	flexor digitorum superficialis
GDP	general dental practitioner
GCS	Glasgow Coma Score
GI	gastrointestinal
HDU	haemodialysis unit
HEMS	helicopter emergency medical services
HIV	human immunodeficiency virus
ICP	intracranial pressure
IM	intramuscular
IPJ	interphalangeal joint
IPPV	intermittent positive-pressure ventilation

ISS	injury severity score
ITU	intensive therapy unit
IV	intravenous
IVI	intravenous infusion
IVRA	intravenous regional anaesthesia
IVU	intravenous urography
JVP	jugular venous pressure
LAD	left anterior descending
MAST	military anti-shock trousers
MCL	medial collateral
MCPJ	meta-carpo phalangeal joint
MI	myocardial infarction
MRI	magnetic resonance imaging
MTOS	major trauma outcome study
NAI	non-accidental injury
NOF	neck of femur
NSAIDs	non-steroidal anti-inflammatory drugs
OPSI	overwhelming post-splenectomy infection
paO_2/CO_2	arterial partial pressure of oxygen/carbon dioxide
PASG	pneumatic anti-shock garment
PAWP	pulmonary artery wedge pressure
PCA	patient-controlled analgesia
PE	pulmonary embolism
PEEP	positive end-expiratory pressure
PIPJ	proximal interphalangeal joint
PPE	personal protection equipment
Ps	probability of survival
PTA	post-traumatic amnesia
PTSD	post-traumatic stress disorder
RICE	rest, ice, compression and elevation
RTA	road-traffic accident
RTS	revised trauma score
SI	sacro-iliac
SIRS	systemic inflammatory response syndrome
SpO_2	pulsed oxygen saturation
SSRIs	selective serotonin re-uptake inhibitors
TBSA	total body surface area
TRTS	triage revised trauma score
TS	trauma score
USS	ultrasound scanning
VF	ventricular fibrillation

PREFACE

The optimal management of the victim of trauma is increasingly recognized as important in its own right and also as a measure of the quality of a hospital's emergency services. Yet the most effective trauma care provision requires not only the co-operation of a wide range of doctors: accident and emergency specialists, trauma and general surgeons, radiologists and anaesthetists, as well as experts in rehabilitation; it also requires the skills of the emergency services, nurses and physiotherapists. Trauma is truly a multi-disciplinary subject. We have tried to bring together in this book a series of trauma related 'key topics' covering a wide range of related specialities. We are grateful to all those experts who have kindly contributed their knowledge and expertise. We hope that this book will allow access to a broad range of information otherwise only found by searching through many specialist volumes and we have tried to make the text readable, pithy and relevant. We have deliberately, therefore, taken the opportunity to include a number of subjects which are uncommon, controversial or the subject of ongoing study.

We hope this book will be helpful to all those involved in the care of the trauma victim, not only doctors, and we would, of course, welcome any comments or criticisms especially with regard to apparent omissions.

Ian Greaves
Keith Porter
Derek Burke

ACKNOWLEDGEMENTS

Our thanks to Ian and Gill Oxley for their expert secretarial assistance (again), to our specialist contributors Sally Bradley, James Briscoe, Chris Constant, Peter Dyer, Mike Elliot, Alasdair Gray and Marcus Green, to our families for their patience during yet another project and finally to Jonathan Ray of BIOS for his support and advice.

To Julia, Sally and Janet
with love

ABDOMINAL INJURIES

Intra-abdominal injuries are a common cause of preventable death from trauma, with ruptured spleen and liver being the most common missed diagnoses. Clinical signs are often subtle, absent or masked by those of other injuries or the effects of alcohol and drugs. The possibility of intra-abdominal trauma should always be considered. Frequent re-evaluation of the patient is required to detect such injuries and early surgical involvement is mandatory.

Anatomy

The abdominal cavity extends from the level of the fourth intercostal space to the pelvis and is divided into three compartments:

The peritoneal cavity This cavity contains the following structures:

- Liver.
- Spleen.
- Jejunum.
- Ileum.
- Transverse colon.
- Sigmoid colon.

The retroperitoneal space The retroperitoneal space contains the following structures:

- Aorta.
- Vena cava.
- Upper renal tracts.
- Duodenum.
- Retroperitoneal parts of the colon.
- Pancreas.

The pelvis The pelvis contains the following structures:

- Iliac vessels.
- Female genitalia.
- Bladder.
- Lower ureters.
- Rectum.

Diagnosis

History Establish the mechanism of the injury, whether it is blunt or penetrating trauma. Locate the site of pain and tenderness.

Examination

This follows the traditional approach of inspection, palpation, percussion and auscultation.

1. Inspection. The patient must be completely undressed and the whole area from the lower chest to the perineum should be examined including the back. During the 'log roll' look for:

- Bruising.
- Abrasions.
- Lacerations.
- Entry or exit wounds.
- Imprint marks.

2. Palpation. Check for:

- Localization of pain.
- Guarding.
- Rebound.
- Crepitus (from underlying fractures to ribs or pelvis).

3. Percussion. Look for rebound tenderness, this can also be elicited by asking the conscious patient to cough.

4. Auscultation. Listen for:

- Bowel sounds.
- Bruits.

5. Rectal examination. Look for:

- Blood (from penetrating bowel injuries).
- Palpable bony fragments (from pelvic fractures).
- Position of the prostate (a high riding prostate suggests a posterior urethral injury).
- Presence and degree of sphincter tone.

Rectal examination is mandatory before inserting a urethral catheter.

6. Vaginal examination. Look for:

- Blood.
- Palpable bony fragments.
- Amniotic fluid.

7. Urethral and perineal examination. Look for evidence of urethral injury:

- Blood at the tip of the urethra.
- Perineal bruising.
- Extravasation of urine.

A positive examination is the best indicator of significant intra-abdominal injury, a negative examination does not exclude such injury and indicates the need for further evaluation.

Investigations

Blood tests

- Cross match/group and save.
- Full blood count.
- Urea and electrolytes.
- Amylase.
- Pregnancy test (if indicated).
- Kleinhauer test (if indicated).

X-ray examination

In addition to the standard films taken for all major trauma cases (lateral c-spine, chest and pelvis) the following may be considered:

1. Plain abdominal film.

- Free air in the abdominal cavity (mandates laparotomy).
- Extraluminal retroperitoneal air (mandates laparotomy).
- Loss of psoas shadow.

2. Contrast studies.

- Urethrography.
- Cystography.
- Upper GI series.
- Lower GI series.
- Intravenous urogram.

Ultrasound

Can identify free intraperitoneal fluid and splenic, hepatic and renal haematomas. It can be used in the resuscitation room, is non-invasive, but it is operator dependent.

CT scan

This requires that the patient be transported to the scanner and is therefore confined to the stable patient. It provides information on the site and extent of intra-abdominal, retroperitoneal and pelvic injuries. It may miss injuries to the hollow viscus.

Diagnostic peritoneal lavage (DPL)

The open method is used, the procedure ideally being carried out by the surgeon looking after the patient. Indications are:

- Equivocal clinical examination.
- Unreliable clinical examination due to:

    (a) Reduced conscious level.
    (b) Influence of alcohol or drugs.
    (c) Neurological impairment (e.g. cervical cord lesion).

Relative contraindications to performing DPL include:

- Previous abdominal surgery.
- Gross obesity.
- Clotting disorders.
- Cirrhosis.
- Pregnancy.

An existing need for laparotomy is the only absolute contraindication for DPL.

1. *Accuracy of DPL.*
- *Sensitivity.* 98% (for intraperitoneal bleeding).
- *False negative rate.* 2% of cases due to injuries of retroperitoneal or pelvic structures or to ruptured diaphragm.
- *False positive rate.* 2% of cases due to bleeding from pelvic fractures, from the operative site or injury to intraperitoneal structures during the procedure.

2. *Indicators of a positive DPL.*

- Red cell count $>100\,000/\text{mm}^3$.
- White cell count $>500/\text{mm}^3$.
- Presence of   bile, bacteria, faecal material.

Complications are uncommon but include:

- Haemorrhage from the operative site.
- Peritonitis from bowel perforation.
- Perforation of the bladder.
- Injury to intra-abdominal or retroperitoneal structures.
- Wound infection.

It must be emphasized that the above mentioned investigations are an adjunct to clinical assessment, the presence of a definite indication for laparotomy should not delay early surgery in order to perform such tests.

Management

Nasogastric/orogastric intubation for aspiration of gastric contents

- This reduces the risk of aspiration.
- Relieves gastric distension (reducing diaphragmatic splinting).
- Inspection for blood (may indicate the presence of upper gastrointestinal injury although nasopharyngeal trauma is the most common cause of gastric blood in this situation).

An orogastric tube should be used if there is suspicion of a basal skull fracture.

Urinary catheter

This can be used for:

- Decompression of the bladder.
- Continuous monitoring of urine output.
- Inspection and testing of urine for blood.

The possibility of urethral injury must be excluded prior to passing a urinary catheter.

Indications for immediate laparotomy

- Hypotension with evidence of abdominal injury.
  (a) gunshot wounds,
  (b) stab wounds,
  (c) blunt trauma with blood on DPL.
- Peritonitis: early or subsequent.
- Recurrent hypotension despite adequate resuscitation.
- Extraluminal air.
- Diaphragmatic injury.
- Intraperitoneal perforation of urinary bladder on cystography.
- CT evidence of injury to the pancreas, gastrointestinal tract, and specific injuries to the liver, spleen and/or kidneys.
- Persistent amylase elevation with abdominal findings.

Further reading

American College of Surgeons Committee on Trauma. Abdominal Trauma. In: *Advanced Trauma Life Support: Program for Physicians*. Chicago: American College of Surgeons, 1993; 141-58.

Robertson C, Redmond AD. *The Management of Major Trauma*. Oxford: Oxford University Press, 1991.

Skinner D, Driscoll P, Earlam R. *ABC of Major Trauma*. London: BMJ Publications, 1991; 46-50.

Related topics of interest

ADULT RESPIRATORY DISTRESS SYNDROME (ARDS)

ARDS is a complex response of the lung to injury, either direct (e.g. aspiration or inhalation of noxious gases) or indirect (e.g. sepsis or pancreatitis). It is characterized by a defect in oxygen diffusion due to filling of the alveoli by a proteinaceous fluid secondary to an increase in vascular permeability not due *primarily* to infection. ARDS is the severe end of a spectrum of acute lung injury with an overall mortality rate of 40%.

Definitions

ARDS is defined by the presence of hypoxia (with a paO_2 to FiO_2 ratio of less than 200), low lung compliance and widespread pulmonary infiltrates on CXR, with a normal pulmonary artery wedge pressure (PAWP). There should be a known precipitant of ARDS. The presence of a raised left atrial pressure should be excluded as there is a well-defined haemodynamic abnormality responsible for hypoxaemia in these cases.

Investigations

The following investigations may be helpful:

1. Plain chest radiograph. The characteristic radiography changes may not appear for several hours after the precipitating insult, thereafter full progression to bilateral infiltrates takes 4–24 hours. The changes may be indistinguishable from those of congestive cardiac failure.

2. CT scan. This reveals patchy involvement of the lung with areas of normal lung tissue. The degree of involvement on the CT scan correlates with the degree of impairment of gas exchange and the compliance.

3. Measurement of gas exchange. Arterial blood gases initially reveal a respiratory alkalosis associated with hypoxaemia. The hypoxaemia is relatively resistant to supplemental oxygen administration and mechanical ventilation becomes necessary. The ratio of paO_2 to FiO_2 correlates with outcome.

4. Bronchoalveolar lavage. As well as being used for diagnosing nosocomial or opportunistic infection, bronchoalveolar lavage will reveal an increase in polymorphs to up to 80% of the total cells (normally <5%). The presence of eosinophils suggests that the patient may respond to steroids.

5. *Haemodynamic monitoring.* Pulmonary oedema, high cardiac output and low pulmonary artery wedge pressure are characteristic but not diagnostic. The main role of haemodynamic monitoring is to exclude cardiogenic pulmonary oedema and to guide fluid administration.

No validated index of lung injury has been described. The cornerstone of diagnosis remains the presentation of progressive hypoxaemia in the presence of pulmonary infiltrates and the absence of evidence for elevated left atrial pressure.

Treatment

There is no specific treatment to correct the underlying vascular permeability or inflammatory process. Treatment is aimed at supporting and maintaining gas exchange, organ perfusion and aerobic metabolism. Therapeutic agents which are believed not to be helpful in ARDS are also briefly reviewed.

1. *Mechanical ventilation.* Mechanical ventilation is indicated when spontaneous ventilation on maximal inspired oxygen concentration fails to maintain an adequate paO_2, although ventilation will often be instituted earlier, based upon the clinical course of the patient. As well as maintaining paO_2, mechanical ventilation reduces the work of breathing and helps to maintain aerobic ventilation. Large tidal volumes and high peak airways pressure may cause lung injury and exacerbate ARDS.

2. *Positive end expiratory pressure (PEEP).* PEEP increases lung volume, prevents alveolar closure and reduces atelectasis, thereby improving oxygen transfer. It does not prevent ARDS in those at risk of developing the syndrome and it may cause barotrauma and reduce cardiac output. There is no evidence that PEEP improves outcome in ARDS.

3. *Extracorporeal membrane oxygenation (ECMO).* A prospective randomized study of ECMO showed no effect on outcome for patients with ARDS.

4. *Intravascular oxygenation.* There are no published data to suggest any clinical benefit from the use of intravascular oxygenation in ARDS.

5. *Positioning of the patient.* Repositioning of the patient with non-uniformly distributed lung infiltrates has been shown to improve oxygenation; however, practical problems exist with nursing patients in, for instance, the prone position.

6. *Fluid management.* Restriction of fluids to maintain a low pulmonary wedge pressure while maintaining cardiac output has been shown to improve pulmonary function and improve outcome.

7. *Drug therapy.*

- Exogenous surfactant. Patients with ARDS have normal levels of surfactant, but it is dysfunctional. Although studies are being carried out, there is no confirmed role for surfactant in clinical treatment at present.
- Corticosteroids. There is evidence that steroids do not alter the outcome of ARDS when used early in the disease. There is some evidence that steroids are of some benefit when used in the fibroproliferative phase of the disease (5–10 days). The few patients with high levels of eosinophils in bronchoalveolar lavage have been shown to benefit from steroids.
- Ketoconazole. Used as a potent inhibitor of thromboxane synthesis and leukotriene biosynthesis, ketoconazole has shown some benefit in preventing ARDS in at-risk patients (sepsis or multiple trauma).
- Nitric oxide. Nitric oxide is a selective pulmonary vasodilator which has been shown to reduce pulmonary artery pressure and intrapulmonary shunting while increasing the ratio of paO_2 to FiO_2 but having no effect on mean arterial pressure or cardiac output. No studies have yet been published to support its use in ARDS.
- Eicosanoids and their inhibitors. Ibuprofen and other prostaglandin-inhibiting non-steroidals and alprostadil (prostaglandin E_1)have not been shown to improve outcome from ARDS.
- Antiendotoxin and anticytokine therapy. Although there is some suggestion that such agents may decrease the incidence ofARDS, none has been shown to reduce mortality.

- Antibiotics. There is no evidence that routine use of antibiotics in the absence of established infection reduces the mortality of ARDS, indeed the routine use of antibitoics on intensive care units has been shown to lead to the emergence of resistant bacteria and make the treatment of established infections more difficult.

Prevention

There is some evidence to suggest that large molecular weight resuscitation fluids, such as starches, may have a preventive effect if used early enough in patients at risk of developing ARDS. Suggested mechanisms include the possibility that these large molecules block holes in capillaries and reduce the consequences of capillary leak, as well as reducing the binding of neutrophils to epithelium and consequent migration through the capillary wall.

Outcome of ARDS

The overall mortality has fallen from 60% to 40% in the past decade; this improvement is probably attributable to improved intensive care rather than any specific modality of treatment. Death usually occurs in the first 2 weeks of illness and is due to sepsis, multiorgan failure or the underlying illness. Common complications during treatment include barotrauma, nosocomial infection and stress-related GI bleed.

Further reading

Kollef MH, Schuster DP. The acute respiratory distress syndrome. *New England Journal of Medicine*, 1995; **332** (1): 27–34.
Treasure T. A surgeons view of adult respiratory distress syndrome. *British Journal of Hospital Medicine*, 1994; **52** (2/3): 108–12.

Related topics of interest

ADVANCED TRAUMA LIFE SUPPORT (ATLS)

The Advanced Trauma Life Support (ATLS) course was devised in the USA in 1978 to provide a systematic approach to the management of major trauma in the first hour, the aim being to maximize the probability of survival. The Royal College of Surgeons of England adopted the course in November 1988 as the standard for management of trauma in the UK. There are four main components to the course:

- Primary survey (ABCs).
- Resuscitation.
- Secondary survey.
- Definitive care.

The course also covers the principles of preparation, triage, post resuscitation monitoring, re-evaluation and inter-hospital transfer.

Primary survey and resuscitation

In practice the primary survey and resuscitation are carried out at the same time. Life-threatening conditions are identified immediately in a sytematic manner and management of these conditions is carried out at the time of their identification. The sequence for identifying life-threatening conditions is based on identifying and managing those which pose the greatest threat to life first. The following sequence is used:

- Airway management and cervical spine control.
- Breathing and ventilation.
- Circulation with control of haemorrhage.
- Disability: neurological status.
- Exposure/environmental control.

Airway management and cervical spine control	The airway should be secured whilst maintaining immobilization of the cervical spine. Cervical spine immobilization can be achieved by manual in-line immobilization, by use of a long spinal board or by using sand bags, tapes and a semi-rigid cervical collar.
Breathing	Adequacy of ventilation should be assessed by inspection, palpation, percussion and auscultation. Conditions which pose an immediate threat to adequate ventilation are identified and treated at this stage. If the patient's breathing is absent or inadequate then artifical ventilation is provided with a bag valve mask device or a mechanical ventilator. All victims of major trauma require supplemental oxygen irrespective of their ventilatory status or blood gas values.
Circulation	Adequacy of blood volume and cardiac output is assessed initially by observing the following:

1. Level of consciousness. Homeostatic mechanisms maintain cerebral perfusion even in the presence of significant hypovolaemia. An altered level of consciousness may indicate marked hypovolaemia.

2. Skin colour. Patients who are warm and pink peripherally rarely have life-threatening hypovolaemia. Conversely those who are peripherally shut down, particularly if young and healthy, have a significant degree of hypovolaemia requiring immediate resuscitation. All victims of major trauma require two large-bore cannulae and blood drawing for cross-match or grouping and save.

3. Pulse. The rate, rhythm and quality should be assessed. The presence of peripheral pulses and contralateral pulses should also be assessed.

Disability (neurological evaluation)

A brief evaluation of the level of consciousness and pupillary size and response should be made. The level of consciousness can be assessed using the AVPU method:

A Alert.
V Responds to verbal stimuli.
P Responds to pain.
U Unresponsive.

Exposure/environmental control

The patient is completely undressed to aid examination. Care should be taken to ensure that the patient does not become hypothermic by maintaining a warm environment, using warm IV fluids and blankets.

During or at the end of the primary survey baseline physiological parameters are recorded:

- BP.
- Pulse.
- Respiratory rate.
- SpO_2.
- Glasgow Coma Score.

Baseline investigations taken at this stage include:

- FBC.
- U&E.
- Arterial blood gases.
- Group and save/cross match.
- ECG.
- Lateral cervical spine X-ray.

- Chest X-ray.
- Pelvic X-ray.

A urinary catheter and nasogastric or orogastric tube should be placed at this stage.

If the patient's condition deteriorates during resuscitation, then a complete re-evaluation is undertaken beginning with airway.

The primary survey should be repeated as often as necessary. Once the patient is stable a decision should be made as to the need for definitive treatment and whether this requires transfer to another unit.

Secondary survey

Following the primary survey and resuscitation and when the patient is stable a complete head-to-toe examination is carried out to look for other injuries. This secondary survey includes re-evaluation of the vital signs.

The secondary survey should include a systematic examination of the following:

- Head and skull.
- Maxillofacial.
- Neck.
- Chest.
- Abdomen.
- Perineum, rectum and vagina.
- Musculoskeletal system.

These should include:

- A complete examination of the patient's back using a 'log-roll' taking care to protect the cervical spine.
- A complete neurological examination.
- Appropriate X-rays based on the findings of the secondary survey.
- Appropriate laboratory investigations.
- Special investigations as required (e.g. peritoneal lavage).
- 'Tubes and fingers in every orifice'.

A detailed history of the mechanism of the injury and relevant patient history should also be taken, the AMPLE history is used:

A   Allergies.
M   Current medications.

P   Past medical history.
L   Last meal.
E   Events/environment related to the injury.

ATLS courses are run regularly at various venues around the country, certification following a course lasts for 4 years after which a shorter re-certification course is taken. Details of forthcoming courses can be obtained from the Royal College of Surgeons of England.

Futher reading

American College of Surgeons Committee on Trauma. Initial assessment and management. In: *Advanced Trauma Life Support: Program for Physicians*. Chicago: American College of Surgeons, 1993; 17–37.

Related topics of interest

Abdominal injuries (p. 1)
Cervical spine injuries (p. 65)
Genitourinary trauma (p. 104)
Imaging (p. 156)
Intravenous fluids (p. 167)
Paediatric aspects of trauma (p. 216)
Pelvic fractures (p. 224)
Pregnancy and trauma (p. 242)
Preventable deaths (p. 246)
Shock (p. 261)
Trauma teams (p. 309)

AEROMEDICAL EVACUATION

The first specialized helicopter ambulance service in the UK was started in Cornwall in 1987. It has been estimated that a single helicopter can cover 8000 square miles within a response time of 20 minutes.

Within the UK aeromedical evacuation can be divided into primary casualty evacuation and secondary patient transfer.

These roles are primarily carried out by helicopters. Fixed wing aircraft also have a role in international repatriation of the sick and injured (air ambulances).

Medical helicopters are currently provided by the Royal Air Force and coastguard (Air Sea Rescue), ambulance services, helicopter emergency medical service (HEMS), and occasionally the police.

Advantages of helicopter transfer

The advantages of primary casualty evacuation by air are:

- Convenient delivery of highly skilled personnel.
- Convenient delivery of specialist equipment.
- Rapid access to conventionally inaccessible sites and inhospitable terrain with winch access to cliffs and water.
- Rapid response times.
- Ease of delivery of patients to appropriate specialist facilities.

Secondary patient transfer by air allows patients suffering from conditions such as burns or spinal injuries to be transferred rapidly from an initial receiving hospital to a specialist centre.

The majority of this work is carried out by helicopters rather than fixed wing aircraft as they do not require a conventional airfield or landing strip. Although both forms of aeromedical evacuation are faster than road travel, the time taken to load or unload the patient must be remembered, and secondary transfers (for example transporting a patient from the helicopter landing site to the receiving hospital by conventional ambulance) will add considerably to transfer times.

Approach to a helicopter

Ideally a helicopter should only be approached once the rotors have stopped and the pilot has given a 'thumbs up' sign. If it is necessary to approach a helicopter with moving rotors, approach on the downhill side, if appropriate duck, and do not carry anything above your head. Never approach a helicopter from the rear because of the risk of injury from the tail rotor.

Disadvantages of helicopter transfer

Helicopters are extremely expensive to operate, they also have a relatively small range compared to fixed wing aircraft (300 miles for a Wessex, 600 miles for a Sea King or Dauphin helicopter).

Other disadvantages include:

- Injury from rotor blades or downdraught.
- Noise (usually greater than 90 decibels and sufficient to cause hearing damage with long-term exposure, necessitating ear defenders and causing communication problems).
- Vibration.
- Flicker.
- Windchill/cold.
- Equipment problems. Medical equipment including defibrillators may interfere with navigational equipment.
- The space available in a helicopter is limited (176 cubic feet of cabin space with 78 cubic feet of storage space in a Dauphin).
- Helicopters require a landing site at least 15 m diameter which is firm, non-sloping and free of debris.
- Air sickness.
- Movement during helicopter transfer is usually less disruptive than that of road transfer, it is however closely related to the development of nausea and sickness in susceptible individuals.

Crew

It has been suggested that the 'ideal' crew for a medical helicopter should consist of two pilots, a paramedic and a doctor. This is the crew currently carried by the HEMS helicopter. The majority of other 'medical' helicopters carry a crew of paramedics and pilots only.

The Civil Aviation Authority (CAA) now recognizes 'medical passengers' who play no part in operating the helicopter during flight, and 'medical crew' who need to be trained in navigation, flight preparation, VHF/RT operation, air-traffic control and meteorology.

International air evacuation

International air evacuation of the sick or injured is usually undertaken either to provide access to better healthcare in the UK than is available in the particular country concerned, or to avoid enormous healthcare costs in foreign countries. Clearly before a patient can be transferred it is essential to establish that the transfer itself would not be detrimental to the patient's health. Administrative problems with such transfers include:

- The importation of controlled drugs.
- The necessity to ensure ambulance facilities for transfer on arrival in the UK.
- The availability of an appropriate hospital bed.

Helicopter and mortality rates

Due largely to its expense, aeromedical evacuation remains controversial and there is currently a desire to demonstrate an effect on mortality. In a limited study, Nicholl *et al.* suggested an improvement in the survival rate for critically injured patients but with no demonstrable improvement over the complete range of patients. The implication that patients with minor injuries fare worse with helicopter evacuation has also been drawn from American data. Nicholl *et al.* compared the HEMS system carrying a doctor with the conventional paramedic-based land ambulance service. It is apparent that more comprehensive studies are required before any definite conclusions can be drawn.

Further reading

Aeromedical evacuation. In: Greaves I, Hodgetts T and Porter K (eds) *A Handbook of Immediate Care*. London: WB Saunders, 1995.

Aeromedical evacuation. In: Greaves I, Hodgetts T and Porter K (eds) *Emergency Care: a Textbook for Paramedics*. London: WB Saunders, 1996.

Nicholl JP, Brazier JE, Snookes HA. Effects of London Helicopter Emergency Medical Service on survival after trauma. *British Medical Journal*, 1995; **311**: 217–22.

Sellwood N. An ambulance helicopter for emergency call. *Archives of Emergency Medicine*, 1992; 280–9.

Related topics of interest

Pneumatic anti-shock garment (PASG/MAST suit) (p. 238)
Preventable deaths (p. 246)
United Kingdom trauma outcomes (p. 315)

AMPUTATION: TRAUMATIC

Upper limb amputation

Major traumatic amputation of the upper limb proximal to the wrist is uncommon. In all cases of upper limb amputation the patient should be considered for re-implantation, and early discussion with the appropriate speciality should be arranged. Where transfer is planned, the amputated part should be wrapped in saline-soaked gauze, placed in a plastic bag and transported with the patient on, but not in direct contact with, ice. Traumatic amputation of the upper limb will not be considered further.

Lower limb amputation

Trauma is the most common cause of lower limb amputation worldwide. The pattern and mechanism of such amputations vary from region to region. In the developed world road-traffic accidents and industrial accidents account for most cases. In most of the developing world this pattern is also found, although in areas where there has been military conflict land mines account for the majority of such injuries.

Early traumatic amputation
This is usually evident on initial presentation, the affected part being partially or completely separated from the proximal limb. The mechanism of injury and state of the limb will determine whether limb salvage is possible. Clean, distal, 'guillotine'-type injuries have a better prognosis for salvage than avulsed, contused proximal injuries.

Late traumatic amputation
The limb may initially appear viable, but amputation is required as a result of the initial injury as a result of:

- Vascular insufficiency secondary to direct arterial injury, secondary thrombosis or compartment syndrome.
- Infection, e.g. gas gangrene.
- Functional impairment, where a salvaged limb proves to be non-functional and impairs rehabilitation.

Management
The initial resuscitation priorities are to identify and treat life-threatening injuries. A major amputation may compromise circulation, in which case attention should be directed to controlling active bleeding. Initially this should consist of direct pressure to the wound. Attempts to probe the wound or to blindly clamp bleeding vessels may

convert a potentially salvageable limb into a non-viable limb.

When the patient has been stabilized, the decision to proceed to early amputation will depend on assessment of the viability of the limb. This may involve other specialists, for example vascular surgeons and plastic surgeons.

1. Vascular. The vascular state is assessed (see key topic: Vascular trauma), if persisting vascular insufficiency is suspected, angiography should be performed to determine the extent and level of the injury and potential for repair.

2. Neurological. Proximal division of major nerves, even with primary repair, has a poor outlook. Degeneration of distal musculature will occur prior to healing of the nerve. Early amputation will allow rehabilitation to begin and will avoid the psychological problems associated with delayed amputation.

3. Soft tissue. If missed, compartment syndrome will lead to necrosis of the muscle of the affected compartments and functional impairment. Commonly associated with tibial fractures, early decompression is required based upon clinical suspicion. Major degloving injuries may not be immediately evident, but may involve deeper tissues and render the distal limb non-viable.

4. Bone. Compound fracture leading to chronic osteomyelitis, or fracture leading to non-union, may be indications for delayed amputation.

Level of amputation

If, for functional reasons or because the limb or part of the limb is non-viable, the decision is made that amputation should proceed, then the decision as to the level of the amputation must be made.

The level of the amputation will be determined by:

- The extent of the initial injury.
- The vascular supply to the limb. This may have been assessed pre-operatively by angiogram. If angiography has not been performed, amputation should be performed at a level where the muscle is healthy and bleeds freely. This will help ensure a healthy, healing stump and allow early mobilization.

AMPUTATION: TRAUMATIC **19**

- The presence of infection, which should be treated prior to amputation if possible. If amputation is to treat infection, then the level of amputation should be proximal to the level of infection. In the specific case of gas gangrene, infection is often present proximal to the obvious level of infection. Radical amputation is indicated in this instance.
- The need to maintain function. The aim of amputation, as well as to save life, must be to maintain as much function in the limb as possible. Distal amputation has a better outcome than more proximal amputation. If possible, the knee joint should be preserved.

The level of amputation may be dictated by the level of the initial injury and may consist merely of trimming the residual stump of a complete amputation. In cases of delayed amputation, a planned procedure may allow time to plan the best functional level.

Post-operative management   Early rehabilitation will improve functional recovery and aid in psychological re-adjustment.

Further reading

Gray DWR. Limb amputation. In: Morris PJ, Maly RA, (eds.) *Oxford Textbook of Surgery*. Oxford: Oxford University Press, 1994; 488–50.
Michaels JA. Major amputations of the lower limb. *Surgery*, 1995; 151–6.

Related topics of interest

Blast injuries (p. 39)
Compartment syndrome (p. 70)
Crush syndrome (p. 74)
Gunshot injuries (p. 112)
Vascular trauma (p. 317)

ANAESTHESIA

Anaesthesia may be needed for multiple injuries, or for trauma to a single body area. Local, regional or general anaesthetic techniques may be used. Anaesthesia should only be practised by those with appropriate training.

Special problems

1. Full stomach. Gastric stasis can be caused by pain or opiates. The stomach may also contain swallowed blood or alcohol.

2. Airway obstruction. This may be due to unconsciousness, foreign bodies, haematoma or oedema. Laryngeal oedema develops rapidly in burn inhalational injury.

3. Cervical spine injury. Neurological deficit may be caused, or worsened, by manipulation for airway management or central line insertion.

4. Impaired ventilation. Caused by head injury (central hypoventilation), chest injury (pneumothorax, haemothorax, flail chest, lung contusion), spinal cord injury (respiratory muscle paralysis) or drugs.

5. Shock. Hypovolaemic, cardiogenic (myocardial contusion, cardiac tamponade), or neurogenic (spinal cord injury with vasodilation) all cause problems. Large volume fluid replacement may be needed, but there is a risk of haemodilution, coagulopathy, pulmonary oedema and increased bleeding.

6. Head injury. Impaired consciousness makes assessment difficult. Raised intracranial pressure (ICP) may be worsened catastrophically by hypoxia, hypercarbia, volatile anaesthetics and intubation. Hypotension lowers cerebral perfusion when ICP is raised.

7. Multiple organ failure. After major trauma the following can occur rapidly:
- Adult respiratory distress syndrome (ARDS).
- Acute renal failure (ARF).
- Disseminated intravascular coagulation (DIC).
- Impaired liver function.
- Systemic inflammatory response syndrome (SIRS).

8. *Medical problems.* These may have led to the original injury (e.g. MI, diabetes, epilepsy), and may remain undetected in the mentally obtunded patient.

9. *Alcohol and drug abuse.* It is known that these lead to trauma, and cause later physiological problems and withdrawal states.

General anaesthetic management of major trauma

Resuscitation

- Airway control; intubation and artificial ventilation if needed (see below); high-percentage oxygen.
- Treatment of chest conditions impairing ventilation (e.g. drainage of pneumothorax or haemothorax).
- Large-bore venous access (two or more 14G IV cannulae); adequate fluid resuscitation.

Investigations

- Chest, cervical spine and pelvic X-rays as appropriate.
- Baseline full blood count, urea and electrolytes.
- Cross-matching: adequate amounts of blood, with fresh frozen plasma and platelets available for major bleeding.
- Arterial blood gases for all major trauma, particularly in head or chest injury, or previous lung disease.
- ECG if age $\geq$ 50 years, chest trauma, or suspected heart disease.

Induction

Intubation

- Rapid sequence induction and oral intubation is usual using pre-oxygenation and cricoid pressure to prevent pulmonary aspiration. Manual in-line cervical spine stabilization allows the cervical collar to be removed temporarily, or mouth opening will be limited.
- Blind nasal intubation (recommended by ATLS teaching in the unconscious spontaneously-breathing patient, to minimize neck movement. However when performed by a competent anaesthetist, oral intubation is generally considered at least as safe and is preferred in the UK).
- Awake fibreoptic intubation may be safest in suspected cervical spine injury or airway obstruction, if the expertise is available.

Induction agents	• Etomidate: cardiovascularly stable; often used for the shocked patient. • Thiopentone and propofol: cause more hypotension (may be severe in hypovolaemia). • Ketamine (see p. 173): sometimes used for the shocked patient. Causes hypertension and tachycardia. Raises ICP. *NB. contraindicated in head injury.*
Muscle relaxants	• Suxamethonium: allows the quickest and safest intubation. Justified in head injury despite raising ICP. Raises intra-ocular pressure (relatively contraindicated in perforating eye injury). Contraindicated in major burns after the first 48 hours due to severe hyperkalaemia (also reported after prolonged immobility following trauma).
Maintenance	Intermittent positive-pressure ventilation (IPPV) is usual, with oxygen, nitrous oxide, a muscle relaxant, opiate and a volatile anaesthetic. Non-steroidal anti-inflammatory drugs add to analgesia, but impair renal function and worsen bleeding in major trauma.

1. Nitrous oxide is avoided in:

• Undrained pneumothorax, or pneumomediastinum.
• Head injury with aerocele.
• Suspected air embolism.

Nitrous oxide diffuses into closed air-containing spaces, causing expansion.

2. In head injury:

• Hyperventilate to a $pCO_2 \approx 4kPa$, to promote mild cerebral vasoconstriction, and reduce ICP (effective only for 12–24 hours).
• Avoid hypotension and hypoxia.
• Use minimal or no volatile agent (isoflurane ≤ 1MAC causes least rise in ICP).

3. General considerations.

• Monitoring: in addition to routine, consider temperature, urine output, arterial and central venous pressure monitoring, and Swan–Ganz catheterization.

| | • | Temperature maintenance: (e.g. heated mattress or blanket) to reduce vasoconstriction, preserve cardiac function and minimize coagulopathy. |
| | • | Fluid/blood transfusion: consider a warmed rapid transfusion system; monitor coagulation status; give blood, clotting factors and calcium as needed; allow for additional losses (e.g. burn oedema); avoid excessive crystalloids in head or chest injury. |

Post-operative care

1. Analgesia.

- Opiate infusions.
- Patient-controlled analgesia.
- NSAIDs.
- Local anaesthetic techniques.

2. Need for intensive or high-dependency care.

Ketamine

Ketamine is a 'dissociative analgesic', which can be used as a general anaesthetic, or for analgesia in sub-anaesthetic doses. It is used for short procedures (e.g. change of burns, dressings, and in pre-hospital care; see Ketamine, p. 173).

Further reading

Clark RSJ, Carson IW. Anaesthesia for trauma and shock In: Nunn JF, Utting JE, Brown BR Jr (eds) *General Anaesthesia*, 5th Edn. London: Butterworths, 1989; 686–95.

Giesecke AH, Rylah LTA. Anaesthesia for the burned patient. In: Nunn JF, Utting JE, Brown BR Jr (eds) *General Anaesthesia*, 5th Edn. London: Butterworths, 1989; 958–65.

Illingworth KA, Simpson KH. *Anaesthesia and Analgesia in Emergency Medicine*. Oxford: Oxford University Press, 1994; 3–246.

Related topics of interest

ANALGESIA

Pain in acute trauma results from injury to bone and soft tissue, as well as the effects of surgery. As well as relieving pain, analgesia may:

- Minimize sympathetically mediated vasoconstriction and tachycardia.
- Reduce chest complications, in chest or abdominal trauma/surgery.
- Ameliorate the metabolic and hormonal response to pain.

Pain management

This may include:

1. *Immobilization* of fractures and soft-tissue injuries such as:

- Slings, splints or strapping.
- Plaster of Paris.
- Traction.
- Surgical fixation.

2. *Local applications.*

- Cold compresses.
- Cooling of burns, burns dressings.

3. *Drugs* (see below).

- Systemic analgesics (including inhalational analgesia).
- Local/regional anaesthesia.

4. *Psychological* (reassurance and explanation).
Multimodal treatment (i.e. combinations of drugs and other forms of treatment, gives optimal analgesia).

Systemic analgesic drugs

Simple analgesics
(e.g. aspirin and paracetamol)

- Only adequate for mild pain.
- May not be absorbed orally due to gastric stasis.

Entonox®

Cylinders containing 50% oxygen/50% nitrous oxide for inhalation are useful for short painful procedures, (e.g. splinting, and in pre-hospital care).

Advantages:
- Moderate analgesia (equivalent to 10 mg morphine).
- Rapid onset.

- Easy administration (can be given by non-medical personnel).
- Minimal respiratory and cardiovascular depression.
- Self-administration via a demand valve prevents overdose.

Disadvantages:
- Needs patient co-operation.
- Unsuitable for prolonged administration.
- Contraindicated in undrained pneumothorax, pneumomediastinum, or head injury with aerocele (nitrous oxide diffuses into closed, air-containing spaces causing expansion).
- May raise intracranial pressure.
- Causes nausea/light-headedness.
- Nitrous oxide liquefies at $-7°C$, causing separation of contents.

Non-steroidal anti-inflammatory drugs (NSAIDs)

Useful in bony pain and soft tissue inflamation, either alone or in combination with other analgesics.

Advantages:
- Moderately effective.
- No respiratory depression or sedation.
- No nausea or vomiting.
- Opiate-sparing effect when given concurrently.
- Can be given orally, IV, IM or rectally.

Disadvantages:
- May impair renal function, especially in hypovolaemia.
- Prolong bleeding time (reduce platelet aggregation).
  NB. These two features make NSAIDs unsuitable in the acute phase of major trauma.
- Gastrointestinal bleeding.
- Bronchospasm in some asthmatics.

Drugs/doses:
- Diclofenac: 100 mg rectally, 50 mg orally, 75 mg deep IM.
- Ketorolac: starting dose 10 mg orally, IV or IM.

Opiates

These are suitable for moderate to severe pain, they should be titrated IV. Oral or IM administration is unreliable in major trauma, as absorption from gut and muscle is impaired. Naloxone must be available whenever opiates are used.

Advantages:
- Potent analgesia.
- Sedation.

Disadvantages:
- Oversedation possible (unconsciousness in overdose).
- Respiratory depression, or even apnoea. Respiration should be monitored, and oxygen given if needed.
  NB. Hypoxia and hypercarbia may cause a dangerous rise in ICP in head injury.
- Miosis (interferes with assessment of head injury).
- Nausea/vomiting; reduced gut motility.
- Hypotension, especially in hypovolaemia.
- Addiction (very unlikely in the acute setting; this possibility should not deter the use of adequate doses).

Drugs/doses:
- Morphine, diluted and titrated IV: 2–5 mg initially, then 1–2.5 mg increments as required.
- Nalbuphine (may have a 'ceiling' to respiratory depression; used by paramedics): 10–20 mg IV or IM.
- Codeine phosphate (less potent; preferred in head injury): 30–60 mg IM.
- Also give an anti-emetic such as metoclopramide 10 mg IV.

Intravenous infusions are more effective than repeated IM injections for persistent pain. Continued monitoring of respiration is important. A regimen of 1 mg/ml morphine at 1–5 ml/hour is suitable.

Ketamine

A potent analgesic, also used as a general anaesthetic. Used in sub-anaesthetic doses (up to 0.5 mg/kg IV) for painful procedures such as:

- Manipulation/splinting.
- Repeated dressings (e.g. burns).
- Extrication in pre-hospital care.

Patient-controlled analgesia (PCA)

PCA is intermittent, patient-triggered IV administration of pre-set doses of an opiate analgesic, via a specially designed infusion pump. By pushing a button, the patient can trigger bolus doses and titrate his own analgesia. Ideally provided as part of a hospital acute pain service for optimal follow-up and effectiveness.

Pump settings

The following pump settings are pre-set at the start of treatment (figures in brackets are a typical regimen using morphine sulphate):

- Concentration of opiate solution (1 mg/ml).
- Initial bolus dose (5 mg).
- Patient-triggered bolus doses (1 mg).
- Lockout interval (i.e. the period after each bolus during which the pump will not deliver another) 3–5 mins.
- Background infusion rate (1 mg/hour): often not used, as it may increase the risk of respiratory depression without improving analgesia.
- Maximum total dose over a given period (20 mg/4 hour).

Frequent reassessment is needed to ensure these settings are adequate.

Advantages:
- Better, more constant analgesia than intermittent IM injections, with lower total opiate dose.
- Avoids subjective assessment (and underestimation) of the patient's pain by hospital staff.
- No delay between a request for analgesia and drug delivery.
- Psychological benefit to the patient of controlling his own analgesia.
- Avoids repeated IM injections.
- Minimal risk of overdose.

Disadvantages:
- Patient must be alert, co-operative, and understand the technique.
- Special equipment and staff training needed.
- A dedicated IV line is needed, or a T-connector with a one-way valve to prevent opiate back-tracking into other infusions.
- Overdose may occur if other people (e.g. relatives) push the button.

Further reading

Welchew E. *Patient-Controlled Analgesia.* London: BMJ Publishing Group, 1995.

Young Y, Fletcher SJ. Sedation and analgesia for the trauma patient. In: Park GR, Sladen RN (eds). *Sedation and Analgesia in the Critically Ill.* Oxford: Blackwell Science, 1995; 186–208.

Related topics of interest

Entonox® (p. 90)
Ketamine (p. 173)
Local blocks: regional anaesthesia (p. 184)
Splintage (p. 276)
Thoracic and lumbar epidural anaesthesia (p. 292)

ANKLE INJURIES: FRACTURES

Ankle fractures account for 11% of all fractures presenting to the A&E Department and are the most common fracture of a weight-bearing joint. Ankle fractures are common at all ages after childhood during which bony injury is rare. When fractures do occur in children they are usually epiphyseal injuries classified using the Salter–Harris system. The anatomy of the ankle is shown in *Figure 1*.

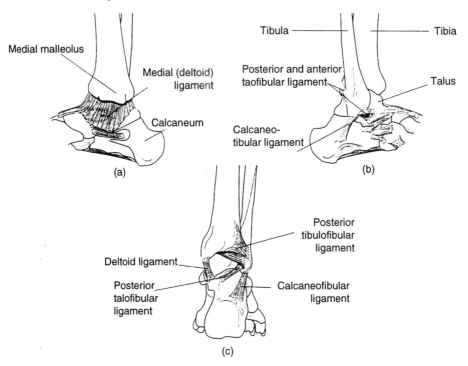

Figure 1. Anatomy of the ankle joint. (a) Medial view, (b) lateral view, (c) posterior view. Reproduced from Greaves, Hodgetts and Porter (eds) (1997) *Emergency Care: a Textbook for Paramedics* with permission from WB Saunders.

Classification

The most commonly used classification is the Lauge–Hanson classification (1948). Double titles are given to each fracture, the first referring to the position of the foot at the time of injury, the second to the direction of movement of the talus within the ankle mortice in response to the applied force. The Lauge–Hanson classification is the most useful classification in terms of prognosis.

- Supination–adduction fractures.
- Supination–eversion (external rotation) fractures.

- Pronation–abduction fractures.
- Pronation–eversion (external rotation) fractures.

Each group of fractures has a number of well-defined stages which occur as the injury progesses: an example (for supination–eversion injury) is given in *Figure 2*. In supination–eversion injury the incidence of secondary osteoarthritis is 2.6% with a stage II injury and 23.6% with a stage IV injury.

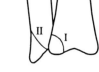

I   Injury to anterior tibiofibular ligament, insubstantial rupture of small bony avulsion

II Oblique fracture at level of joint

III Posterior malleolar fragment

IV Pull off fragment through medial malleolus or deltoid ligament rupture

Figure 2. Supination–eversion injuries.

A more practical classification for use in Accident and Emergency Departments is the Weber classification (1972) which is based on the AO grouping according to the level of the fibular fracture in relation to the tibial articular surface at the ankle joint (plafond).

Type A: fracture below the level of the syndesmosis (the distal tibiofibular joint).

Type B: fracture at the level of the syndesmosis (spiral fractures beginning at the level of the plafond and extending proximally).

Type C: fracture above the level of the syndesmosis.

Type B and C fractures are invariably unstable and may be displaced at the onset or become displaced later. It is these fractures that are likely to need orthopaedic intervention.

Open reduction and internal fixation or conservative management?

In a relatively small series ($n = 47$) Godsiff *et al.* (1993) reported that when comparing internal fixation and early return to movement with plaster of Paris immobilization, the early movement group contained more patients who were completely pain free, returned to work sooner and had no radiological signs of osteoarthrosis. However, the early mobilization group spent longer in hospital (10.2 days compared to 7.4 days in the plaster group). Approximately one-third of all patients complained of some pain at 5 years whether treated operatively or non-operatively. A recent audit of ankle fractures in the elderly has shown that surgery carries acceptable risks providing attention is paid to surgical techniques and fixation is carried out according to the AO manual.

The critical factor in outcome is the quality of the reduction, whether achieved by closed means or open. The greater the number of traumatic lesions (*Figure 2*) the worse the overall prognosis, this reflects the magnitude of the original causative force. If osteoarthrosis is going to occur, it is usually radiologically evident within 18 months of injury.

The most significant correlation between a single lesion from the Lauge–Hanson classification and outcome is the presence of a posterior tibial fracture. Small flake fractures do not contribute to secondary osteoarthrosis, but otherwise, the larger the posterior fragment, the greater the risk of osteoarthrosis. The *talocrural angle* when measured is a reliable indicator of prognosis. This is the angle measured when a perpendicular is dropped from a line through the tibial plafond and intersects the line drawn between the tips of the malleoli in an antero-posterior radiograph. The angle is normally 83° ± 4°. The difference between the two ankles in a normal individual is less than 2°. It is proposed that any degree of fibular shortening or rotation, or both (i.e. non-anatomical reductions) will produce an abnormal angle.

In summary, there is strong evidence and opinion to support the accurate reduction of ankle fractures, as this appears crucial if good results are to be obtained, and in many cases this can only be achieved by operative intervention. However, when considering long-term results and the development of osteoarthritis, there is no conclusive evidence that satisfactory open reduction and internal fixation is better than satisfactory closed manipulation. There is, however, increasing evidence to suggest that less stiffness and pain occurs in patients treated by operation, providing a good reduction is obtained and no operative complication occurs.

Fracture dislocation

- Early reduction reduces associated soft-tissue complications.
- Grade I and grade II open fractures are most commonly seen.
- Neurovascular compromise when present (numbness or lack of pulses) commonly returns to normal following appropriate reduction.
- Emergency reduction in the Accident and Emergency Department may be appropriate.

Operative intervention in common open fractures should not be delayed because of associated injuries in the presence of significant contamination. As with closed fractures, there is a window of opportunity for surgical intervention and fixation. This is usually before 8 hours or after 5–7 days. During the intervening period, the ankle is usually too swollen for definitive surgery. Because of residual swelling and bruising and a risk of operative skin compromise, surgery may occasionally be delayed beyond 10 days.

Further reading

Apley AG and Solomon L. *Apley's System of Orthopaedics and Fractures*, 7th Edn. Oxford: Butterworth Heinemann, 1993.
Godsiff SP *et al.* Fractures of the ankle. *Injury*, 1993; **24** (8): 529–30.

Related topics of interest

ANKLE INJURIES: SPRAINS

Ankle sprains are a common condition in all A&E Departments. Common symptoms include variable degrees of pain, swelling and inability to weight bear. Ninety per cent are lateral ankle sprains, two-thirds of the anterior talofibular ligament (ATFL) and one-third of the calcaneofibular ligament (CFL). In many cases initial examination is too painful to allow specific diagnostic tests.

Diagnosis

Specific tests:

- ATFL: palpation over the sinus tarsi during inversion stress in plantar flexion.
- CFL: inversion stress in plantar flexion.

The anterior drawer test is used to assess instability of the ankle joint. With the ankle in mid plantar flexion, the tibia is stabilized and the hind foot drawn forwards. Anterior subluxation of the talus under the tibia indicates ATFL incompetence. Talofibular incompetence may not be detected in the acute phase but may be recognized in patients with persisting symptoms or recurrent sprains.

Investigation

X-ray investigation to exclude bony injury is required if there is:

- Bony tenderness around the posterior edge or the tip of the lateral malleolus (distal 6 cm of the fibula).
- Bony tenderness around the posterior edge or the tip of the medial malleolus (distal 6 cm of the tibia).
- An inability to weight bear both immediately and in the emergency department.

These guidelines are taken from the Ottawa Rules, compliance with which may reduce the X-ray rate in ankle sprain by as much as 25%. X-rays may, however, be necessary if the patient has an altered level of consciousness due to alcohol, drugs or severe associated injuries. X-rays will also be required if the patient has altered lower limb sensation (for example from a spinal injury) or if the swelling is so gross as to prevent palpation for specific tenderness. All patients should be advised to attend for review if pain or inability to weight bear have not begun to improve after 5 days.

Treatment

Treatment is non-operative in the vast majority of sprains and includes **R**est, **I**ce **C**ompression and **E**levation (**RICE**).

Plaster of Paris immobilization may be rquired for the symptomatic relief of severe sprains. Operative intervention may be indicated in young high-calibre athletes and specific referral to a sports injury clinic may be appropriate. Outcome following ankle sprain is improved by appropriate physiotherapy.

Recurrent ankle sprain or chronic lateral ankle sprain requires further investigation by inversion stress films in dorsiflexion and plantar flexion with consideration of surgical stabilization by tenodesis.

Further reading

Apley AG and Solomon L. *Apley's System of Orthopaedics and Fractures*, 7th Edn. Oxford: Butterworth Heinemann, 1993.

Steill I *et al*. A multicentre trial to introduce the Ottawa Rules for use of radiography in ankle sprains. *British Medical Journal*, 1995; **311:** 592–7.

Related topics of interest

ANTIBIOTIC THERAPY

The number of prescriptions for antibiotics rank second only to prescriptions for analgesics in the A&E Department. Common indications for prescribing them include:

- Treatment of an established infection with a known organism (either cultured or known pattern of infection).
- Treatment of an established infection with an unknown organism (blind therapy).

Prophylaxis

Patterns of prescribing vary from department to department. The most common reason for prescribing is prophylaxis in wound management. Such liberal use of antibiotics should, however, not replace adequate wound management, the priorities of which are:

- Early vigorous cleaning.
- Adequate debridement.
- Tetanus prophylaxis.
- Immobilization.
- Elevation.

Such management in the absence of antibiotics often results in wound healing without infection, absence of wound management but prescription of antibiotics usually results in wound infection.

It is not always necessary to obtain microbiological samples prior to prescription, particularly when the likely organism in an established infection is known (e.g. *Staphlococcus aureus* or *β*-haemolytic streptococci in soft tissue infections), or when the local pattern of organisms in uncomplicated infections is known (e.g. specific organisms and patterns of resistance in uncomplicated urinary tract infection). In such instances the microbiology department will usually circulate lists of 'best guess' antibiotics for use in specific infections. Regular sampling of the local pattern of organisms and sensitivities is required to ensure that the current recommended antibiotics provide adequate cover.

Factors in deciding which drug to prescribe

1. Patient factors.

- History of drug allergy.
- Renal function.
- Hepatic function.
- Resistance to infection (e.g. whether immuno-compromised).
- Ability to tolerate the drug by oral route.

- Severity of illness.
- Ethnic origin.
- Possibility of pregnancy.
- Whether breast feeding.
- Whether taking oral contraception.

2. *Pathogen.*

- Known or likely organism.
- Antibiotic sensitivity of pathogen.
- Site of infection.

3. *Drug factors.*

- Local restrictions in prescribing.
- Cost.
- Side effects.
- Contraindications.
- Duration of therapy.

Recommended antibiotics

Recommended drugs for a wide range of specific infections can be found in the current issue of the *British National Formulary* (BNF) as well as a list of infections for which prophylaxis is considered useful.

Specific traumatic conditions

Generally agreed antibiotics for specific traumatic conditions include:

1. *Penetrating trauma to the lower gut.*

- IV cefuroxime and metronidazole.

2. *Penetrating trauma to the upper gut.*

- IV cefuroxime.

3. *Compound fractures.*

- IV cefuroxime.

4. *Prevention of gas gangrene.*

- IV benzylpenicillin or IV metronidazole.

5. *Human bites* (particularly to the hand).

- Oral/IV augmentin.

6. *Other soft tissue injuries.*

- Oral flucloxacillin or erythromycin.

Further reading

British National Formulary. London: BMA/Royal Pharmaceutical Society of Great Britain.

Related topics of interest

HIV infection (p. 143)
Human and animal bites (p. 147)
Tetanus and gas gangrene (p. 286)

BLAST INJURIES

An explosive is a substance which undergoes chemical decomposition into gaseous products at high pressure and temperature.

- Low explosives burn on ignition and only explode if confined (petrol, gunpowder).
- High explosives do not require confinement, but need the use of a detonator (TNT, Semtex).

Physiology

1. Shock wave. The rapid expansion of hot gases produces a shock wave travelling at high speed (> 3000 m/sec) with an instantaneous rise to peak pressure (the overpressure). The overpressure falls as the speed of the shock wave falls ending as a phase of negative pressure.

In conventional explosions the overpressure lasts about 1 msec, the negative phase ten times as long. The shock wave travels more rapidly in media denser than air and is reinforced after reflections from solid surfaces due to summation of incident and reflected waves. The release of energy is inversely proportional to the square of the distance from the epicentre.

$$E \propto \frac{1}{D^2}$$

2. Blast wind. Behind the shock wave is an area of turbulence known as the 'blast wind' producing a dynamic pressure causing direct injury and converting fragments into potentially lethal high speed missiles.

Injuries due to blast

Primary

The overpressure associated with the shock (or blast) wave is responsible for the primary blast injuries, the mechanisms of which are:

1. Compression. Direct compression of the victims body.

2. Spalling. Disruption of the more dense tissue at interfaces of tissues of different density and air/fluid interfaces (eyes, lungs, bowel).

3. Shear waves. Shearing forces along tissue planes due to tissues of different densities being set in motion relative to each other. This produces submucosal and subserosal haemorrhages.

4. *Implosion.* Air compressed and heated by the shock wave re-expands with explosive force causing rupture of the tympanum, bowel or lung.

Examples of specific injuries are as follows:

(a) Ear damage. Blast damage may result in:
   - tympanic membrane rupture,
   - disruption of the ossicles,
   - inner ear damage.

   The usual symptoms are tinnitus and deafness.

   Orientation of the ear relative to the shock wave is important in determining whether ear damage will occur. An overpressure of approximately 100 kPa will rupture a healthy eardrum.

(b) Injury to abdominal organs. Rarer in explosions in air than explosions underwater. Injuries include:
   - bowel contusions,
   - multiple perforations,
   - frank gastrointestinal haemorrhage.

(c) Lung contusion (blast lung). Blast lung is rare occurring in less than 10% of survivors. Usually mild it may take the form of rapidly progressive respiratory distress syndrome. Lung contusions occur with haemorrhage, non-cardiac pulmonary oedema and the opening up of pulmonary arterio-venous fistulae.

   An overpressure of 175 kPa will produce blast lung (overpressure of 300 kPa will produce structural damage to buildings). Generally pure blast effects are more marked with military rather than terrorist bombs, unless the latter contain very large amounts of explosive.

(d) Sudden death. Blast overpressure may occasionally result in sudden death with no apparent evidence of external injury. This is believed to be due to cerebral or coronary artery embolism although fatal dysrhythmias have also been suggested.

Secondary

In dealing with the victims of an explosion, the most significant injuries are usually those caused by fragments – secondary blast injuries. The fragments are produced by the blast wave and propelled by the blast wind.

- *Primary fragments.* Fragments of the explosive device itself (bomb casing, nails, ball-bearings).
- *Secondary fragments.* Fragments of building or furniture (glass, masonry or wood).

All fragments can be assumed to be heavily contaminated with bacteria.

Tertiary

Tertiary blast injuries are caused by the blast wind. Victims may be thrown through the air sustaining impact injuries particularly to solid organs. Such injuries have been estimated to occur in 25% of the victims of an explosion in a confined space. Traumatic amputations occur as parts of the body are torn off. The bodies of victims very close to the explosion may be completely disrupted. Tertiary injuries may also result from building collapse. Crush injuries result from falling masonry. Rarely, in prolonged entrapment, amputation at scene may be required.

Burns

- *Flash burns.* These occur at the moment of impact affecting exposed parts of the body. Although the appearance of such burns may be dramatic they are usually superficial. Airway oedema and destruction may occur.
- *Flame burns* may occur if surrounding buildings ignite exacerbating inhalational injuries from smoke and hot gases.

Psychological problems

Approximately 40% of those involved in a bomb incident will develop psychological sequelae. Psychological problems appear less troublesome amongst trained rescue personnel, especially if their actions had a beneficial result.

Treatment of blast injuries

- All those suspected of having been exposed to a significant blast effect should be observed in hospital.
- Any patient with a ruptured eardrum should be considered to have been exposed to a significant blast effect and observed appropriately.
- Blast lung may not occur for up to 48 hours following injury (normal 6–12 hours) hence the need for close observation. Mandatory chest X-ray (CXR) reveals bilateral diffuse shadowing with hypoxia and hypercardia on blood gas analysis.
- It has been suggested that intermittant positive pressure ventilation (IPPV) and positive end expiratory pressure (PEEP) should be avoided in the first hour following blast injury due to the risk of air embolism. Because of the risk of pneumothorax consideration should be given to the insertion of bilateral prophylactic chest drains. Vigorous chest

physiotherapy is required during the severe phase of shock lung. The role of corticosteroids remains controversial.

- Over enthusiastic infusion of crystalloids may exacerbate pulmonary oedema. Where possible resuscitation should be with colloids or blood.

- The majority of uncomplicated tympanic perforations recover with conservative treatment.

- Following significant blast injury, many patients develop diffuse mild abdominal pains due to multiple small haemorrhages, conservative treatment is appropriate. However, if the patient develops any sign of peritonitis, significant gastrointestinal haemorrhage (a nasogastric tube should be passed) or shows free gas on (mandatory) abdominal X-ray (AXR), a laparotomy should be performed.

- Unlike 'guillotine' amputations, traumatic amputations caused by blast winds are avulsive with the amputated part being torn away from the body. Nerves and tendons are often avulsed at a proximal level and reimplantation is rarely, if ever, possible. Surgery is confined to toilet with extensive debridement of dead and potentially infected tissue.

Further reading

Blast and gunshot injury. In: Greaves I, Dyer P, Porter K (eds). *A Handbook of Immediate Care*. London: W B Saunders, 1995.

Greaves I, Porter K (eds). *Blast and Gunshot Injuries in Prehospital Medicine: the Principles and Practise of Immediate Care*. London: Arnold, 1997.

Kirby NG, Blackburn G (eds). *Field Surgery Pocket Book*. London: HMSO, 1981.

Ryan J, Cooper G (eds). *Ballistic Trauma*. London: Arnold, 1997.

Related topics of interest

Amputation: traumatic (p. 18)
Gunshot injuries (p. 112)
Penetrating cardiac injury (p. 229)
Psychological aspects of trauma (p. 249)
Tetanus and gas gangrene (p. 286)

BLUNT CARDIAC TRAUMA

Blunt cardiac injuries are relatively common. Biffl *et al.* (1994) reported a 30% incidence of cardiac contusion in high-risk blunt trauma victims and Wisner *et al.* (1990) reported cardiac contusion in 14% of victims of immediate death from blunt trauma. Injury may be direct (for example, a blow from a steering wheel to the chest) producing contusion at the site of impact, or indirect due to an acute rise in intracardiac pressure producing tears and contusions away from the site of impact. However, the prognosis is good, and the majority of patients recover fully without any evidence of long-term problems.

Pathophysiology

The histology of cardiac contusion is broadly similar to that of myocardial infarction. Specific differences include:

- More haemorrhages.
- A distinct boundary between normal and abnormal myocardium.
- Changes are usually epicardial changes, although intramural or transmural extension may occur.
- The area of injury is unrelated to the areas supplied by the coronary vessels, and reflects only the area of dissipated force.
- Changes are not precipitated by coronary spasm or coronary artery occlusion.
- Being retrosternal, the right ventricle is the more common chamber injured.

On microscopic examination, there are areas of patchy necrosis, oedema and haemorrhage. These local areas of injury result in arterio-venous shunting and, correspondingly, a fall in right ventricular contractility and a rise in right ventricular end-diastolic pressure. This produces a shift of the intraventricular septum to the left with reduction in left ventricular pre-load and compliance. Left ventricular failure may occur.

Diagnosis

The possibility of a patient having suffered a blunt cardiac injury should arise from the history, and information obtained from the emergency services can be invaluable. However, such a history may not be available in the multiply injured or unconscious casualty, and a high index of suspicion should therefore be maintained.

1. Physical signs. Anterior chest wall tenderness and bruising are suggestive of significant force having been applied to the chest. Pattern bruising from steering wheel markings may occur. Fracture of the sternum is a marker of high-energy transfer injury.

2. Electrocardiographic abnormalities. In a meta-analysis of 12 prospective studies Christenson and Suton (1993) reported ECG abnormalities in 33% of patients. No specific abnormality was consistently detected. Abnormalities included:

- ventricular dysrhythmias;
- atrial fibrillation;
- bundle branch block.

Since the right ventricle is most commonly injured, due to anatomical positioning, the ECG, which predominantly reflects left ventricular changes, is not reliable. ECG abnormalities therefore contribute to the diagnosis of, but are not themselves diagnostic of, cardiac contusion.

Seventy-eight per cent of those patients who develop arrythmias do so within 24 hours and 91% within 48 hours (Fabian *et al.*, 1991). Patients with a previous history of heart disease are at particular risk of developing arrythmias.

3. Cardiac enzymes. Christenson and Suton reported that CPK-MB elevation is non-specific, and cannot be used to predict cardiac complications (see also Biffl *et al.*, 1994; Fabian *et al.*, 1991).

4. Echocardiography. Trans-thoracic echocardiography provides a very sensitive diagnostic tool. Studies using this technique have shown ventricular wall motion abnormalities in up to 25% of blunt chest wall injuries (Helling *et al.*, 1989; Reif *et al.*, 1990). Trans-thoracic echocardiography may be of help in the selection of those patients who require observation on an intensive care unit (Reif *et al.*, 1990).

Trans-oesophageal echocardiography may provide information in blunt cardiac injury when trans-thoracic echocardiography is unhelpful (usually for technical reasons), and it will also assist in the diagnosis of any associated thoracic aortic injury (Shapiro *et al.*, 1991). Trans-oesophageal echocardiography may therefore be considered the most sensitive investigation in blunt cardiac trauma.

Treatment

In the majority of cases no specific management other than careful observation is required. Treatment is indicated if there is compromised cardiac function, with or without arrythmias. Treatment options include reducing right ventricular afterload, inotropic support, cardiac pacing, and (rarely) the intra-aortic balloon pump.

Further reading

Biffl WL, *et al*. Cardiac enzymes are irrelevant in the patient with suspected myocardial contusion. *American Journal of Surgery,* 1994; **169:** 523.

Christenson MA, Suton KR. Myocardial contusion: new concepts in diagnosis and management. *American Journal of Critical Care,* 1993; **2:** 28.

Fabian TC, *et al*. A prospective evaluation of myocardial contusion: correlation of significant arrythmias and cardiac output with CPK-MB measurement. *Journal of Trauma,* 1991; **31:** 653.

Helling T , Dale P, Beggs CW, Grouse LJ. A prospective evaluation of 68 patients suffering blunt chest for evidence of cardiac injury. *Journal of Trauma,* 1989; **29:** 361.

Reif S, Justice JL, Olsen WR, Prager RL. Selective monitoring of patients with blunt cardiac injury. *Annals of Thoracic Surgery,* 1990; **50:** 530.

Roxburgh JC. Review: myocardial contusion. *Injury,* 1996; **27:** 603–5.

Shapiro MJ, *et al*. Cardiac evaluation in blunt thoracic trauma using trans-oesophageal echocardiography. *Journal of Trauma,* 1991; **31:** 835.

Wisner DH, Reed WH, Riddick RS. Suspected myocardial contusion: triage and indications for monitoring. *Annals of Surgery,* 1990; **212:** 82.

Related topics of interest

BRACHIAL PLEXUS INJURIES

Although uncommon, brachial plexus injuries can be devastating, occurring as they most commonly do in young active people as a consequence of motorcycle accidents.

Anatomy (*Figure 1*)

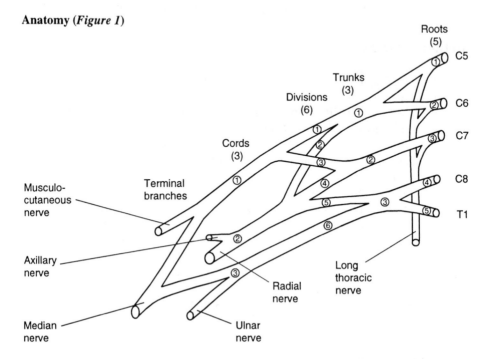

Figure 1. Anatomy of the brachial plexus.

The nerve supply to the upper limb is derived from the anterior primary rami of the C5 to T1 nerve roots via the brachial plexus. The plexus is composed of:

- Five roots (C5 to T1), which enter the upper part of the posterior triangle of the neck by passing between scalenus anterior and scalenus medius muscles.
- Three trunks (upper, middle and lower), which traverse the posterior triangle. The upper trunk is predominantly formed by the C5 and C6 roots, the middle trunk is formed predominantly by the C7 root and the lower trunk by the C8 and T1 roots.
- Six divisions (three anterior and three posterior), which split from the trunks behind the clavicle, one anterior and posterior division deriving from each trunk.

- Three cords (lateral, posterior and medial), formed by the combination of the divisions in the axilla. The names of the individual cords reflecting their relationship to the axillary artery as they embrace it. The anterior division of the upper trunk continues as the lateral cord, the three posterior divisions combine to form the posterior cord and the anterior divisions of the lower two trunks combine to form the medial cord.

Mechanisms of injury

1. Traction. The classical injury is a traction injury between the head and shoulder sustained by a motorcylist thrown from his motorcycle, resulting in lesions of the upper roots. Traction is also the mechanism of brachial plexus injuries at birth (affecting either the upper or lower trunk).

2. Compression. Classically the 'Saturday night palsy' when a drunk falls asleep with the arm draped over the back of a chair. Pressure on the radial nerve in the axilla results in a wrist drop. This lesion may also be caused by pressure from incorrect use of axillary crutches ('crutch palsy')

3. Laceration. Uncommon in the UK, this can result in injury to single nerves or produce a more complex picture of injury.

Pattern of injury

1. Supraclavicular lesions. Supraclavicular injuries may involve an individual trunk (usually the upper or lower), producing a pattern of neurological deficit characteristic of the trunk involved, the upper two trunks or all three trunks.

- Isolated upper trunk (C5 and C6) lesions cause loss of abduction, external rotation and flexion at the shoulder, combined with loss of flexion and supination of the forearm. The arm hangs limply at the side with the elbow pronated and palm facing backwards (Erb–Duchenne paralysis).
- Combined upper and middle trunk (C5, C6 and C7) lesions cause loss of extension at the elbow, wrist and digits in addition to the deficits caused by isolated upper trunk lesions.
- Isolated lower trunk lesions lead to loss of function of the intrinsic muscles of the hand combined with loss of flexion of the fingers. Such a lesion may result from upward traction on the arm in a breech delivery.

BRACHIAL PLEXUS INJURIES **47**

The hand appears clawed due to the unopposed action of the long flexors and extensors; the metacarpophalangeal joints are extended, with flexion of the interphalangeal joints. An associated Horner's syndrome may result from traction on the cervical sympathetic chain.

- Lesions of all three trunks cause total loss of function of the upper limb.

2. *Infraclavicular lesions.* These injuries are commonly a result of local trauma to the shoulder region, either in isolation or associated with multisystem trauma. Such injuries may be associated with injury to the bony skeleton of the shoulder region, axillary artery or thorax and its contents. Lesions of individual nerves (radial, median, musculocutaneous or axillary nerves) occur either in isolation or in combination.

Diagnosis

Brachial plexus injuries occurring as a complication of major trauma may not be diagnosed in the early stages. This may be due to a combination of factors: the presence of immediately life-threatening injuries may preclude full assessment of the patient initially; clinical signs may be obscured by, or attributed to, associated soft-tissue or skeletal injuries; clinical signs may not be evident or may be difficult to elicit in the obtunded patient.

When such injuries are suspected, either because of clinical signs or evidence of trauma to the shoulder region, a careful, systematic, clinical examination should identify the pathways affected and the level of the injury. Such examination may be combined with electrophysiological investigations.

If vascular injury is suspected, an arteriogram will identify the site and extent of injury.

Types of injury

See chapter on peripheral nerve injuries.

Investigations

The following investigations may be helpful:

- Electrophysiological studies: to identify the nerves affected and the level of the lesion.
- Plain X-rays: to identify co-existing bony injury.
- Arteriography: to identify vascular injury.
- CT scanning with intrathecal contrast: absence of rootlets suggests avulsion (better than myelography).

Management

Management of such injuries requires the early input of an experienced hand surgeon to determine the need for, and timing of, operative intervention after immediately life-threatening injuries have been treated or excluded.

Discontinuities in nerve trunks are repaired using nerve grafts (the sural nerve being the most commonly used graft), fibrin glue is used in preference to suturing to join the ends.

Total avulsion of the nerve roots of the brachial plexus resulting in a useless arm may require amputation.

Prognosis

The prognosis for regeneration after repair is determined by:

- The patient's age: the younger the patient the better the outlook.
- The time from injury to repair: early repair has a better outcome, although the presence of more immediately life-threatening injuries in the presence of recognized brachial plexus injury may preclude early repair.
- The distance between the lesion and end organ. The greater the distance, the poorer the outcome.
- Lesions involving avulsion of the nerve roots are irreparable.

Further reading

Burge P. Injuries of the brachial plexus. *Surgery,* 1990; 2007–11.
Narakas A. Brachial plexus surgery. *Orthopedic Clinics of North America,* 1981; **12:** 303–23.

Related topics of interest

Cervical spine injuries (p. 65)
Hand injuries (p. 116)
Peripheral nerve injuries (p. 234)
Shoulder injuries (p. 265)

BRAINSTEM DEATH AND ORGAN TRANSPLANTATION

Potential organ donors may be divided into two groups:

- Heart beating donors: solid organs.
- Non-heart beating donors: tissues, corneas, heart valves, skin and joints.

Clearly brainstem death tests will only be required in the first group. Corneas may be removed from non-heart beating donors up to 12 hours after death, heart valves, skin and bone up to 48 hours.

Eligibility and exclusion criteria

The decision to remove organs should be taken by two senior clinicians of which at least one (and preferably both) should be a consultant.

Exclusion criteria include:

- Systemic infections.
- History or suspicion of hepatitis (or liver disease), TB or sexually transmitted diseases.
- Malignant disease (except primary brain tumours).
- Renal disease including chronic hypertension and recent urinary infection or patients who have suffered renal anoxic damage (kidney donors).
- Severe atherosclerosis (kidney donors).
- Evidence of high-risk status for HIV infection.
- Dementia.
- Conditions of uncertain aetiology where there is suspected immuno-incompetence or viral involvement:
  - (a) Creutzfeld-Jakob's disease.
  - (b) Multiple sclerosis.
  - (c) Leukaemia.
  - (d) Huntingdon's disease.
  - (e) Clinical immunosuppression.
  - (f) Recipients of human growth hormone.

Contraindications to corneal donation include eye disease or intraocular injury, and children (children's corneas are too thin).

Different acceptable donor age ranges apply to potential donors of different organs, advice can be obtained from the transplant co-ordinator.

If there is any doubt regarding the suitability of a donor, the case should be discussed with the local transplant team or transplant co-ordinator.

Potential donors include those who have suffered severe and irreversible brain damage and those dependent on artificial ventilation or shortly expected to become so.

Consent

If the potential donor carries a signed donor card or has otherwise recorded his/her wish to be an organ donor, there is *no legal requirement* to seek the permission of relatives or to establish their lack of objection, although it is good practice to do so. Permission should be sought from one relative who may be asked if he believes any other relatives would object. If there appear to be no relatives, it is not necessary to carry out attempts to discover them. Relatives' lack of objection need not be confirmed in writing.

There is no major religious group in the UK which objects to organ donation and transplantation. Orthodox Jews, Muslims, Hindus and Christian Scientists believe that organ donation is acceptable only if the donor himself has requested it before death. Although they object to blood transfusion, Jehovah's Witnesses believe that donating or receiving organs is a matter about which each member of the sect must decide for himself. Any member of any of these religions who has not left clear evidence of his willingness to be a donor should be assumed to object to donation and transplantation.

The coroner need not be contacted prior to organ harvesting unless there is any possibility that an inquest will be required, in which case his permission will be required before organs can be removed.

It is appropriate and acceptable to take extra blood for tests, such as tissue typing, when blood is taken for tests directly concerned with the patient's own care. Such tests will also include blood grouping and virology. Other investigations will depend on the organs being harvested (e.g. endotracheal aspiration for culture in heart–lung donors) and appropriate advice should be sought.

Diagnosis of brainstem death

Brainstem tests should be carried out, separately or together, by two doctors, one a consultant and the other a consultant or senior registrar. Neither doctor may be a member of the transplant team. Diagnosis should not normally be considered until at least 6 hours after the onset of coma or if cardiac arrest was the cause of coma, until 24 hours after the restoration of circulation.

To be eligible for brainstem death testing, none of the following may be present:

- Hypothermia $< 35°C$.

- Drugs (narcotics, hypnotics, tranquillizers, neuromuscular blockers, anaesthetic drugs).
- Metabolic and endocrine factors (e.g. diabetes, mellitus, uraemia, Addison's disease, hepatic encephalopathy, thyroid disease).
- Biochemical and acid base abnormality (serum electrolytes, acid base balance and blood glucose).
- Severe hypotension.

In addition the patient must be apnoeic requiring ventilation and suffering from irreversible brain damage of known cause.

The diagnostic tests for the confirmation of brain death are:

1. *Pupils.* The pupils are fixed and do not respond to light (II nerve and sympathetic outflow).

2. *Corneal reflex.* Absent (V and VII nerves).

3. *Vestibulo-ocular reflexes.* No nystagmus occurs following injection of 30 ml of ice cold water into each external auditory canal. The ear drums must be visualized before this test (VIII nerve and brainstem).

4. *Gag reflex.* No gag reflex or reflex response to bronchial stimulation (cough reflex) by a suction catheter passed down the trachea (IX and X nerves).

5. *Absence of motor responses* within the cranial nerve distribution when elicited by adequate stimulation of any somatic area.

6. *Apnoea test.* Following ventilation with 100% oxygen the ventilator is disconnected and oxygen administered at 6 l/min for 10 min or until the $PaCO_2$ rises above the threshold for stimulation of respiration. No respiratory effort should be seen. The test should be monitored using blood gas analysis and particular care is needed with patients with pre-existing respiratory insufficiency.

Once a patient has been certified dead, there is no legal or clinical objection to the administration of any drugs necessary to maintain the optimum condition of the organs (for example desmopressin may be given for secondary diabetes insipidus).

The harvesting operation usually takes 2–4 hours depending on the organs being recovered. Muscle relaxants may be required to overcome abdominal muscle spasm from spinal reflexes.

Further reading

Cadavenic Organs for Transplantation: a Code of Practise Including the Diagnosis of Brainstem Death. Health Departments of Great Britain and Northern Ireland, 1983.
Criteria for the diagnosis of brain stem death. *Journal of the Royal College of Physicians*, 1995; **29:** 381–2.

Related topics of interest

BURNS

Burns comprise approximately 1% of the workload of a general A&E Department, the majority being managed without referral to a regional burns unit (less than 10% of cases require such referral). Burn injury causes about 700 deaths per annum in the UK, the most vulnerable groups being the very young and very old.

The extent and depth of any burn is related to the temperature of the burning agent, the contact time and the anatomical extent of exposure.

Types of burn injury

Scalds
These are burn injuries due to contact with a hot fluid. They are the most common cause of admission for burn injury in the UK and usually occur in the domestic setting; the victims are most often children.

Contact burns
A burn injury due to contact with a hot object, e.g. a radiator or bar fire. Such injuries commonly occur in the domestic setting. The mechanism of injury is of prolonged contact with the hot object, usually in a person who is unable to move either as a result of injury (e.g. the elderly after a fall), or altered conscious level (e.g. epileptics or alcoholics).

Flame injury
This is commonly a result of the ignition of clothing and may occur in patients of any age. The injury most often occurs at home, but may also occur in the industrial setting (e.g. ignition of volatile substances).

Electrical injury
The depth and extent of electrical injury is determined by the current type (AC/DC), the voltage and the presence of an arc or flash component to the burn which sets the clothes alight.

1. Domestic contact burn. This will produce a localized burn of varying depth. The victim who has survived the initial shock can usually be followed up as an out-patient as long as the following criteria have been satisfied:

- There was no significant loss of consciousness.
- There are no ischaemic changes on the ECG.
- The are no arrhythmias.
- The patient does not have a pacemaker.
- There is no exit point.

2. *Conduction burns.* This type of burn may occur in the industrial or domestic setting. The current is conducted through the tissues of the body from the entry point to an exit point. Heating of the tissues occurs in proportion to the resistance to current flow. Early death may occur as a result of VF arrest. Rhabdomyolysis may proceed to renal failure in severe cases.

3. *High-voltage burns.* Such injuries are commonly fatal at the scene of injury. The current flow is accompanied by a thudding sound and a blue flash and the victim may be lifted bodily and thrown for some distance. Early death may occur as a result of paralysis of respiratory muscles (for up to 30 min), VF or asystolic arrest. The survivor may suffer significant physical trauma (including cervical spine injury) and extensive burns due to ignition of clothing. Direct current is characteristically associated with asystolic arrest, indirect current with VF arrest.

Chemical burns

Occur in the domestic and industrial setting. Strong alkalis and acids being the principal agents. Such burns are characterized by progression of the burn due to retention of the injurious agent on the skin.

Burns involving the respiratory tract

Such injuries result from exposure to hot gases and/or toxic products of combustion. The deleterious effects result from a combination of burn injury, principally to the upper airways, and toxicity due to inhalation of, principally, cyanide and carbon monoxide.

Classification of burns

Burns may be classified in two ways, either on the depth of burn (superficial dermal, deep dermal or full thickness, erythema is excluded) or on the need for referral to a regional burns unit (major, intermediate and minor).

Depth of burn

1. *Simple erythema.* Simple erythema is a superficial burn without skin loss, such as occurs in sun burn. The skin is red and tender, but heals in 5–10 days. Simple erythema is not included when calculating the area of a burn.

2. *Superficial dermal (superficial partial-thickness).* The skin is red and painful with thin-walled blisters. Local oedema develops some time after the injury. The germinal layer is not involved and therefore complete healing will occur, usually after 10–20 days.

3. Deep dermal (deep partial-thickness). The skin is white in patches with red mottling and decreased sensation. Healing is by migration of cells from the edge of the burn and takes 25–60 days, with scarring and contracture. (Excision and early grafting is usually performed.)

4. Full thickness. The skin is dry, like leather or charred, there is no pain sensation.The full thickness of the skin and a variable amount of deeper tissues are destroyed. (Skin grafting or flap repair will be required.)

Classification on need for referral

1. Major burns. Such burns have a high mortality and require early referral to a regional unit after initial resuscitation. They comprise all burns of more than 30% of body surface area (BSA) or any burn associated with an inhalational injury.

2. Intermediate burns. Such burns have an expectation of low mortality if treated correctly and may require early surgery. They comprise all burns involving 15–30% of BSA for adults, or 10–30% of BSA for children.

3. Minor burns. Any burn not meeting the above criteria and not involving specific body zones may be managed locally. Burns to the following specified zones should be referred to the specialist burns unit:

- Hands.
- Feet.
- Perineum.
- Face.
- Circumferential limb burns.

Some apparently minor burns may require referral because of problems with nursing care, e.g. in the very young, or in the elderly confused or incontinent.

Management

The initial phase of management of burns follows that of any injury, namely the ABCDE approach. Following exclusion or treatment of any other significant injury, the burn is assessed.

Risk to the airway

The initial assessment of the burn must always address the question, 'Does the airway require immediate protection?'. This may result from obvious airway compromise characterized by features of impending airway obstruction:

- hoarse voice;
- stridor;
- respiratory distress;
- oropharyngeal oedema;
- full-thickness facial burns.

  or by features of respiratory failure:

- inability to speak due to dyspnoea;
- sweating;
- exhaustion;
- tachycardia;
- tachypnoea;
- blood gas analysis: $paCO_2 > 6$ kPa, $paO_2 < 8$ kPa despite maximal O_2 therapy.

Any or all of these features indicates the need for urgent intubation. The victim may not be in obvious respiratory embarrassment at the time of assessment, but several features will indicate the need for possible prophylactic intubation because of the risk that pulmonary injury has occurred. These include:

- History of fire in an enclosed space.
- Altered conscious level.
- Cough, bronchospasm and/or bronchorrhoea.
- Sooty sputum.
- Facial burns.
- Singed nasal hairs.
- Auscultatory sing in the chest.
- Lobar collapse from a soot plug.
- Laboratory evidence of inhalation of toxic gases (raised carboxyhaemoglobin level, metabolic acidosis).

Failure to secure an adequate airway under controlled conditions when the airway is patent may result in inability to secure an airway when respiratory failure and airway obstruction develop due to burn oedema. The onset of such oedema may be rapid and dramatic.

Extent of burn

The extent of the burn can be supplied by mapping it on to a Lund and Browder chart (*Figure 1*). Alternatively the simpler 'rule of nines' can be used (the areas of different parts of the adult body are assessed as follows: head 9%, arms 9% each, front of torso 18%, back of torso 18%, legs 18% each and external genitalia 1%). *The palm and closed fingers of the victim's hand may be considered to represent 1% of the body surface area.*

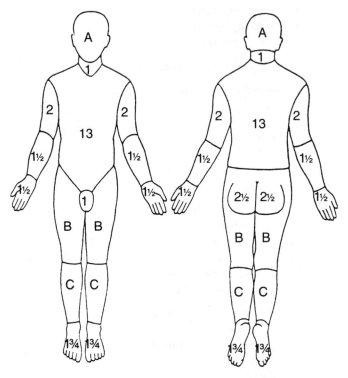

Relative percentage of body surface area affected by growth

Area	Age (years)					
	0	1	5	10	15	Adult
A = ½ of head	9½	8½	6½	5½	4½	3½
B = ½ of one thigh	2¾	3¼	4	4½	4½	4¾
C = ½ of one leg	2½	2½	2¾	3	3¼	3½

Figure 1. Lund and Browder chart. Reproduced from Parr and Craft (1994) *Resuscitation: key data,* 2nd Edn. BIOS Scientific Publishers.

Erythema is ignored and burns are divided into partial-thickness loss and full-thickness loss (deep dermal burns may initially be difficult to assess and may be classified as full or partial-thickness).

It is important to realize that the initial assessment of extent and depth is a guide only. Later reassessment may give an entirely different figure for two reasons:

- Erythema may be assessed as partial-thickness burn, leading to an initial overestimation of burn area compared to when the area is reassessed later after erythema has resolved (typically within 24 hours).
- Partial-thickness burn prior to blister formation may be assessed as erythema, leading to an underestimation of burn area when the area is reassessed later and blistering has occurred.

Progression of burn depth A superficial burn may progress to a deeper burn either from failure to remove the injurious agent (e.g. chemical burns), infection or natural progression of the burn over the first few days.

Management of the burn

After assessment of the burn, the area should be covered with sterile theatre drapes or 'cling film' to prevent heat loss and protect the burn. Creams and ointments should be avoided if victims are to be transferred to a burns unit as their use will make reassessment of the burn difficult.

Fluid resuscitation Several fluid resuscitation regimens are available, with almost every burns unit using its own variation.

The principles of fluid resuscitation in the early stage of a burn are simple. After initial resuscitation to restore circulating volume for any associated injury, the factors determining fluid requirements in the burn victim are:

1. Burn area. The degree of fluid loss is directly proportional to the absolute area of the burn. The absolute area of the burn is calculated from the total body surface area (derived from weight and height, although in practice all formulae use weight only) and the percentage of that area burned.

2. Time elapsed since burn injury occurred. The main loss of fluid from a burn occurs within the first few hours and falls progressively as time elapses. This is the principle behind 'burn periods'. Burn periods are the time intervals in which the calculated fluid requirement is administered, in general the duration of the burn period increases as the time from burn elapses, therefore the fluid volume administered per hour decreases as time from burn elapses.

3. The replacement fluid used. The volume of crystalloid required for replacement is in the region of two to three times the volume of colloid. The specific fluid used depends on availability and local preference.

4. Calculating fluid replacement. The following formulae calculate replacement for burn loss only, replacement for insensible losses should be calculated in addition to this. All formulae are calculated from the time of injury not from the time of presentation to hospital, a period of catching up for significant elapsed time may be required.

(a) Muir and Barclay formula (the standard UK method):

Plasma	0.5 ml/kg/% total body surface area (TBSA) per period
Albumin	0.65 ml/kg/% TBSA per period
Periods in the first 36 hours are	3 × 4 hours 2 × 6 hours 1 × 12 hours

(b) Baxter/Parkland formula

Lactated Ringer's	4 ml/kg/% TBSA per period
Periods in the first 24 hours	50% of total volume in first 8 hours 50% of total volume in next 16 hours
Periods in the second 24 hours	2 litres 5% dextrose plus 0.5 ml/kg/% TBSA as colloid

It should be emphasized that these formulae provide only an estimate of fluid requirements. This should be tailored to the individual patient, based upon repeated reassessment of burn area, haemodynamic response and clinical, biochemical and haematological parameters (urine output, haematocrit, urea).

Full-thickness burns of greater than 10% TBSA will require blood. A fall in haemoglobin may occur in the first few days and should be monitored and replaced with packed cells as required.

Analgesia

Intravenous opiates are the analgesia of choice for extensive burns, they should be given by the intravenous route and given regularly as required.

Infection prophylaxis

Routine use of 'prophylactic' antibiotics is not warranted, giving rise as they do to selection of resistant strains. Infections should be treated on the clinical state of the wound and patient and based upon sensitivities.

Tetanus prophylaxis should be considered for all patients, based upon current guidelines.

Surgical treatment

Skin grafting or, if the deficit is deep enough, formation of a free flap will be necessary in the majority of deep dermal and full-thickness burns.

Outcome

The outcome from burn injury is determined by the depth and extent of the burn, the patient's age and the presence of co-existing disease and concomitant inhalational injury. An approximate percentage probability of dying from a specific burn (without an associated inhalation injury) can be obtained by adding the area of burn to the patient's age. An associated inhalational injury will increase the probability of dying.

Further reading

American College of Surgeons Committee on Trauma. *Advanced Trauma Life Support.* Chicago: American College of Surgeons,1993; 245–59.
Britto J, Phipps A. Major burn trauma: pathophysiology and early management. *Surgery*, 1995; 283–8.
Robertson C, Fenton O. ABC of major trauma. *British Medical Journal*, 1990; **301:** 282–6.
Settle JAD. *Burns – The First Five Days*. Smith and Nephew, 1986.

Related topics of interest

Adult respiratory distress syndrome (ARDS) (p. 7)
Blast injuries (p. 39)
Capnography (p. 62)
Metabolic response to trauma (p. 198)
Pulse oximetry (p. 258)

CAPNOGRAPHY

The capnogram gives a continuous breath by breath recording of the concentration of carbon dioxide in the expired air, this is shown as a dynamic waveform. Machines producing such a display are called capnographs.

The capnometer is a device which displays a numerical concentration of expired (end-tidal) carbon dioxide concentration ($ETCO_2$) and minimum CO_2 concentration during a cycle. The end-tidal CO_2 is the CO_2 concentration at the end of expiration and is generally the maximal CO_2 level measured during the cycle.

Method of action

There are two methods of sampling expired CO_2. The fundamental working of both machines is the same, the only difference is in how the machine displays the concentration of CO_2.

Interpretation of the capnograph waveform requires some skill and in the general setting a capnometer is all that is required.

Different models of capnometers use different techniques for determining the display value. Some display single breath by breath variation in $ETCO_2$ and minimum CO_2 concentration in the cycle, others average the display value over several breaths.

The two methods of sampling expired CO_2 are:

- Side-stream sampling: a small tube is placed within the anaesthetic circuit and draws off a constant stream of expired air into the machine and to the sensor. The disadvantage of such an arrangement is that gas is lost from the circuit and there is a delay, typically several seconds, between the sample being obtained and the result being displayed.

- In-line detectors: in this system the detector is fitted across a clear plastic tube within the anaesthetic circuit. No gas is removed from the circuit and the reading is virtually instantaneous (typically a few tenths of a millisecond from the sample passing the detector through the circuit to the reading being displayed).

The modern portable capnograph uses the principle of infrared absorption spectrophotometry to measure CO_2 concentration. Light from an infrared source is split. One beam is shone through the sample gas, the second is shone through a reference cell containing a known concentration of CO_2. A rotating disc contains a hole to allow the sample light through and a solid area to stop any sample light passing, this acts as a zero reference. By measuring the difference in absorption of infrared light between the sample light source and the reference light source, the concentration of CO_2 is calculated. Various other gases, such as nitrous oxide and water vapour, absorb infrared light and allowances are made for this.

Under ideal circumstances the $ETCO_2$ shows a close correlation with the $paCO_2$, the normal gradient being 0.7 kPa (5 mmHg). The following reduce the accuracy of correlation between $ETCO_2$ and $paCO_2$:

- Tachypnoea.
- Chronic lung disease.
- Hypotension.
- Hypothermia.

If the patient is in a steady state, an initial measurement of simultaneous $ETCO_2$ and $paCO_2$ (by arterial sampling) will indicate the gradient for that patient, and the $ETCO_2$ can then be used to track the $paCO_2$.

Uses of the capnograph

- Confirmation of correct placement of the endotracheal tube in intubation.
- To indicate integrity of an anaesthetic circuit (disconnections, gas leaks, obstruction, etc.).
- Monitoring adequacy of ventilation in the intubated patient.
- To detect rebreathing.
- To indicate air, fat or pulmonary embolism.
- As an apnoea alarm.
- Detection of malignant hyperthermia.
- As an aid to blind nasal intubation.
- Maintenance of a specific $paCO_2$ level (e.g. in the head-injured patient).
- To indicate the adequacy of CPR.
- As a prognostic indicator in CPR (under evaluation).

Note: some of the information listed above can only be derived by analysis of the waveform of a capnograph.

The EASY CAP disposable end-tidal CO_2 detector, is a one-use disposable CO_2 detector. It consists of a plastic casing designed to fit into a standard anaesthetic circuit. An indicator paper changes colour when exposed to CO_2, the colour varying from purple when exposed to room air to yellow when exposed to 4% CO_2. It gives a breath by breath value for $ETCO_2$ and is used to confirm endotracheal tube placement. It is of limited value for confirming tube position in a cardiac arrest situation.

Further reading

O'Flaherty D. *Capnography*. Principles and Practice Series. London: BMJ Publishing Group, 1994.

Related topics of interest

Anaesthesia (p. 21)
Entonox® (p. 90)
Invasive monitoring (p. 170)
Pulse oximetry (p. 258)

CERVICAL SPINE INJURIES

Cervical spine injury occurs in approximately 5–10% of cases of blunt major trauma. Bony injury to the spine may occur in the absence of neurological impairment and conversely neurological impairment may occur in the absence of bony injury. Because of the frequency of cervical spine injury and the consequences of such injury, it is a basic principle of trauma management that all patients suffering major trauma are assumed to have a cervical spine injury until proven otherwise. Therefore all patients falling into this category should have their neck completely immobilized until the cervical spine is cleared. Such immobilization can be achieved by use of a long spinal board or semi-rigid collar, tape and sand bags.

History

Mechanism of injury will suggest the pattern of injuries likely to be encountered. The presence of neurological signs and progression of such signs will suggest the likely site and severity of the injury. Features suggesting the likelihood of having a cervical spine injury include:

- Any injury above the clavicle.
- Any head injury resulting in loss of consciousness.
- Any *high-speed* vehicular injury.

Examination

The patient, immobilized as discussed above, is examined in a neutral position. It is important to emphasize that a semi-rigid collar alone is inadequate to immobilize the cervical spine. Examination of the back of the patient is carried out during the 'log-roll' position. The conscious patient will usually be able to identify the site of local bone tenderness and the level at which sensation is lost. In the unconscious patient the following suggest a cervical spine injury:

- Flaccid areflexia with flaccid rectal sphincter.
- Diaphragmatic breathing.
- Grimacing to pain above but not below the clavicle.
- Ability to flex but not extend at the elbow.
- Hypotension and bradycardia in the absence of hypovolaemia.
- Priapism.

1. Vertebral assessment. Inspection of the spine for evidence of bruising or deformity and palpation for localized tenderness and a 'step-off' deformity can be achieved with the patient partially log-rolled. This requires a four man team, three to manipulate the patient and one to direct the team and remove the long spinal board. To minimize untoward movement of the patient, a complete examination of the back should be performed during the log-roll.

2. *Neurological assessment.* An assessment of motor, sensation, proprioception and autonomic function is made.

- *Motor.* In the conscious patient motor function is assessed by voluntary contraction of specific muscle groups on request. In the unconscious patient involuntary movement to pain is assessed. The response on both sides of the body to paired muscle groups is assessed. Motor function is mediated by the ipsilateral corticospinal tracts in the posterolateral aspect of the cord.
- *Sensation.* In the conscious patient sensation is assessed by the ability to localize pin pricks in specific dematomes. In the unconscious patient sensation is assessed by the response to a painful stimulus. The response is checked in equivalent areas on both sides of the body. Pain and temperature sensation is mediated by the contralateral spinothalamic tract in the anterolateral part of the cord.
- *Proprioception.* This can only be assessed in the conscious patient, by noting the position of the fingers or toes with the eyes closed. The ability to distinguish vibration from a tuning fork can also be used.
- *Autonomic function.* Autonomic function is assessed by the presence or absence of bladder and rectal control and priapism.

Complete and incomplete lesions

The outcome from spinal cord injury depends on whether the lesion is complete or incomplete. Although it may take a considerable period of time to determine how much recovery will occur, the presence of any neurological function at the initial assessment indicates an incomplete lesion. The following indicate an incomplete lesion:

- The presence of superficial pain, elicited by pin prick, or deep pain. Both are mediated by the lateral columns.
- The presence of light touch. Mediated by the posterior and lateral columns.
- Sacral sparing. The presence of sensation in the anal, perianal or scrotal area. It may also be indicated by the presence of voluntary anal contraction.

Clinical features of spinal cord injury

1. Neurogenic shock. Disruption of the descending sympathetic pathways causes loss of sympathetic innervation to the heart, which leads to bradycardia, and relaxation of the peripheral blood vessels, resulting in increased vascular volume and hypotension. The combination of hypotension and bradycardia indicate the possibility of neurogenic shock. The shock often responds incompletely to fluid resuscitation and may require vasopressor agents. Aggressive attempts to fluid resuscitate neurogenic shock can lead to fluid overload. Indications for treating the features of neurogenic shock include:

- Bradycardia: pulse less than 50/min (treat with atropine).
- Hypotension: systolic pressure less than 80 mmHg (treat with inotropes).
- Inadequate urine output (fluids and/or inotropes, use central venous pressure (CVP) monitoring).

2. Spinal shock. An apparent loss of all cord function immediately after injury which results in flaccidity, and loss of reflexes. After an interval, varying from days to weeks, the spinal shock disappears and in areas of the body supplied by parts of the cord with no residual function, spasticity replaces the flaccidity.

3. Abnormal breathing. The effect depends on the level of the lesion. Paralysis of the diaphragm results from lesions involving the C3–C5 region of the cord. Paralysis of the intercostal muscles results from lower cervical or upper thoracic lesions. Both types of lesion result in abdominal breathing and the use of accessory muscles of respiration.

4. Masking of clinical signs. Reduced or absent pain sensation may mask pathology in other areas such as an acute abdomen.

Investigations

A cross-table lateral cervical spine X-ray is taken in all cases of major trauma. Approximately 85% of cervical spine injuries will show up on such a view. The X-ray must include the whole region from the base of the skull to the body of T1. It may be necessary to pull the patient's arms down to get an adequate view or failing that to obtain a swimmer's view. It has been suggested that if the initial lateral film fails to show the upper third of C7, arm traction is unlikely to demonstrate the C7/T1 junction (< 15% of cases).

Even if the cross-table cervical spine view is normal a full set of cervical spine X-rays including antero-posterior (AP) peg view and oblique films are required. A CT scan may be necessary, particularly if bony fragments within the spinal canal are suspected.

Treatment

All patients with a cervical spine injury require expert assessment and should be immobilized until reviewed. Intravenous fluids should be given with care in the presence of neurogenic shock, central venous monitoring may be required. The use of steroids is controversial and should be discussed early with the person who is to take over the definitive care of the patient. If used they should be given within 8 hours of injury.

Spinal cord injury in children

Spinal cord injury occurs less commonly in children than adults and comprises approximately 5% of all spinal injuries. Two-thirds of children suffering from a spinal cord injury have a normal cervical spine X-ray. Therefore a case of a child suspected of having a cervical spine injury, even with normal cervical spine views should be discussed with the appropriate specialist.

Anatomical differences between an adult's and a child's cervical spine include:

- Interspinous ligaments and joint capsules are more flexible.
- The uncinate articulations are poorly developed and incomplete.
- Vertebral bodies are wedged anteriorly and have a tendency to slide forward with flexion.
- The facet joints are flat.

Radiological features of note in the paediatric cervical spine X-ray include:

- Anterior displacement (pseudosubluxation) of C2 or C3 (less common in C3–C4) in 40% of the under seven age group and in 20% of the under sixteen age group
- In 20% of children there is an increased gap between the dens and anterior arch of C1.

- Basal odontoid epiphysis may resemble fracture in under fives, apical odontoid epiphysis may resemble fracture between the ages of five and eleven.
- Secondary ossification centre at tip of spinous processes may resemble a fracture.

Further reading

American College of Surgeons Committee on Trauma. Abdominal trauma. In: *Advanced Trauma Life Support: Program for Physicians.* Chicago: American College of Surgeons, 1993; 141–58.

Ohiorenoya D, *et al.* Cervical spine imaging in trauma patients: a simple scheme of rationalising arm traction using zonal divisions of the vertebral bodies. *Journal of Accident and Emergency Medicine*, 1996; **13:** 175–6.

Skinner D, Driscoll P, Earlam R. *ABC of Major Trauma.* London: BMJ Publications, 1991; 46–50.

Related topics of interest

Advanced Trauma Life Support (ATLS) (p. 11)
Head injuries (p. 124)
Imaging (p. 156)
Laryngeal fractures (p. 183)
Thoracic trauma (p. 295)
Whiplash injuries (p. 321)

COMPARTMENT SYNDROME

Compartment syndrome arises from an increase in the compartmental pressure of a muscle or group of muscles which, if left untreated, progresses to muscle ischaemia, necrosis and ultimately contracture.

Acute compartment syndrome

The syndrome when affecting a particular muscle group or groups is characterized by:

- Increasing rest pain in excess of that expected for the particular injury.
- A feeling of increased tension in the affected compartment.
- Tenderness to palpation.
- Pain on passive stretching of the muscle group (characteristic).
- Decreased sensation or tingling in the distribution of the nerves traversing the compartment.
- Weakness of the affected muscle group.
- Decreased capillary refill.

It is important to remember that the neurological deficit and prolonged capillary refill time are late signs and treatment should not be delayed if they are absent. Peripheral pulses are often present in the acute phase of the syndrome.

Mechanism

The underlying mechanism is an increase in pressure in a non-distensible musculo-fascial compartment. The primary precipitating factor may be a reduction in volume of the affected compartment, or increase in pressure within the compartment.

1. *Reduction in volume.* This may be due to:

- Application of a tight fitting plaster or bandage. This in combination with swelling due to an underlying fracture or soft tissue injury will lead to a rise in pressure in the compartments covered by the constriction.
- Circumferential burns on a limb combined with secondary burn oedema can result in reduced volume due to scar formation and contraction.

2. *Increase in pressure.* Increase in the fluid content of the compartment sufficient to exceed its maximum distensible volume leads to a rise in pressure in the

compartment. The fluid is usually a combination of blood and another factor:

- Burns.
- Fractures.
- Crush injury.
- Acute muscle tears.
- Post-arterial surgery reperfusion injury.
- Bleeding diathesis.
- Release of a surgical tourniquet.
- Pressure due to prolonged general anaesthesia.
- Snake bite.

Site

The following anatomical sites are prone to compartment syndrome:

- Lower leg.
- Forearm.
- Foot.
- Hand.

Compartment syndrome has also been described in the following muscle groups:

- Quadriceps.
- Hamstrings.
- Tensor fascia lata.
- Gluteal muscles.
- Biceps.

Diagnosis

This is essentially clinical. The signs and symptoms described above should lead the diagnostician to suspect compartment syndrome and thus start early treatment.

If the diagnosis is in doubt, the following tests may be carried out:

- Measurement of oxygen saturation distal to the suspect compartment. This may be normal in the early stages.
- Doppler ultrasound to detect reduction in blood flow.
- Measurement of compartmental pressure.

Treatment

Removal of any compressive dressings. Splitting plasters down to the skin. In early cases this may result in a significant reduction in pressure and clinical improvement. Careful observation may obviate the need for fasciotomy.

For established compartment syndrome or early compartment syndrome which fails to respond to conservative measures the following steps should be undertaken:

1. Early surgery. Wide extensive fasciotomy is required including skin, subcutaneous tissue and deep fascia for the entire length of all the compartments involved and with debridement of any necrotic muscle.

2. Generally the wound should be left open. A second look and further debridement of any residual necrotic tissue should be performed when swelling has subsided, generally at 3–7 days. At this stage delayed primary suture or skin grafting may be performed.

3. Measurement of intra-compartment pressures. Indications for urgent fasciotomy include:

- Compartment pressure above 50 mmHg.
- A rise in compartment pressure to within 30 mmHg of diastolic pressure.

It should be emphasized however that fasciotomy should not be delayed while awaiting confirmatory tests once a clinical diagnosis of established compartment syndrome is made.

Chronic compartment syndrome

This classically presents in a young sportsman or woman after a period of exercise. Pain in the affected compartment occurs soon after the onset of exercise and does not settle until some time after exercise has finished, in some cases up to several days later. The diagnosis can be confirmed by measuring compartment pressures at rest and after exercise. Differential diagnoses include:

- Stress fracture.
- Medial tibial stress syndrome.
- Intermittent claudication.
- Popliteal artery entrapment.

The diagnosis is often not considered until other conditions, particularly stress fracture, have been excluded. Treatment is by decompression of the affected compartment. A recurrence rate of 20% is due to incomplete surgery or regrowth of the deep fascia.

Further reading

Gulli B, Templeman D. Compartment syndrome of the lower extremity. *Orthopaedic Clinics of North America*, 1994; **25**(4): 677–84.

Hutson MA. *Sports Enzymes*, 2nd Edn. Oxford: Oxford University Press, 1996.

Related topics of interest

CRUSH SYNDROME

Usually seen in disasters such as earthquakes and other civil disturbances, crush syndrome is rare in the UK, although it may be seen in prolonged entrapment with crush injury. It is also seen very occasionally in alcoholics and drug abusers who have lain on a limb during a period of prolonged unconsciousness. Crush injury due to prolonged application of a tourniquet should not be forgotten. The sinister implications of crush injury arise from the frequent failure of medical staff to recognize the condition early enough.

Pathology

Crushed muscle produces acid myohaematin which blocks renal tubules and leads to renal failure. Toxic metabolites produce profound tissue acidosis and on release may produce cardiac arrest. Electrolyte and acid–base imbalance is followed by disseminated intravascular coagulopathy. The mortality rate is high.

Clinical features

Features in the affected limb:

- Loss of pulses.
- Loss of sensation.
- Reduction or loss of muscle power.
- Redness, swelling and blistering.
- Compartment syndrome.

Systemic manifestations:

- Hypovolaemia.
- Myohaemoglobinuria.
- Progressive renal failure.
- Compartment syndrome may exist as part of a multisystem injury.

Treatment

1. Pre-hospital. Priorities of care follow the ABCDE protocols. A limb that has been severely crushed for several hours should be amputated at the scene. Amputation should be carried out above the level of the crush injury. Once the limb has been released, amputation is valueless in preventing the systemic effects of the muscle breakdown.

2. Hospital management. ABCDE protocols are continued with vigorous fluid resuscitation. Urine output is maximized with diuretics (e.g. mannitol). Maximalization of urine output should not be delayed until the onset of myoglobinuria. Any limb on which a tourniquet has been *in situ* for more than 6 hours should be amputated. In less severe cases, compartment pressures should be monitored. Amputation may reduce the incidence of septic complications.

Further reading

Michaelson M. Crush injury and crush syndrome. *World Journal of Surgery*, 1992; **16**(5): 899–903.

Related topics of interest

Amputation: traumatic (p. 18)
Blast injuries (p. 39)
Compartment syndrome (p. 70)
Diaphragmatic injuries (p. 80)
Intravenous fluids (p. 167)
Metabolic response to trauma (p. 198)
Pelvic fractures (p. 224)
Pneumatic anti-shock garment (PASG/MAST suit) (p. 238)

DENTAL TRAUMA

Injury to the teeth is a common cause of presentation to the A&E Department, either as an isolated injury or as part of more extensive maxillofacial trauma or major trauma. Rarely life threatening, inadequate inital management of such injuries may lead to disfigurement and is a common reason for litigation. Most A&E departments now have ready access to on-call dental or maxillofacial specialists, and it is the duty of the A&E doctor to determine which injuries require intervention by such specialists. The aim of this chapter is to identify those injuries requiring immediate intervention and those which may safely be referred electively.

Terminology

Referral to a specialist is facilitated by proper use of nomenclature. The following summarizes a common method of uniquely naming each tooth.

1. *Primary (deciduous) teeth.* There are 20 primary teeth, these are divided into four quadrants, the upper arch left and right and the lower arch left and right. The primary teeth are sequentially lettered, a to e, from the midline in each quadrant. The teeth are visualized from face on:

Right upper	e	d	c	b	a	a	b	c	d	e	Left upper
Right lower	e	d	c	b	a	a	b	c	d	e	Left lower

e.g.

c | the upper right quadrant canine

| e the lower left quadrant second molar

The primary teeth are named as follows (approximate eruption time):

a	Central incisor	(6 months)
b	Lateral incisor	(9 months)
c	Canine	(18 months)
d	First molar	(12 months)
e	Second molar	(24 months)

2. *Permanent teeth.* There are 32 permanent teeth. Like the primary teeth, they are divided into four quadrants. The permanent teeth are sequentially numbered 1 to 8 from the midline in each quadrant, again visualized face on.

Right upper	8 7 6 5 4 3 2 1	1 2 3 4 5 6 7 8	Left upper
Right lower	8 7 6 5 4 3 2 1	1 2 3 4 5 6 7 8	Left lower

e.g.

2 | the upper right quadrant lateral incisor

| 5   the lower left quadrant 2nd premolar

The permanent teeth are named as follows (approximate eruption dates)

1	Central incisor	(6–7 years)
2	Lateral incisor	(8 years)
3	Canine	(11 years)
4	First premolar	(9 years)
5	Second premolar	(10 years)
6	First molar	(6 years)
7	Second molar	(12 years)
8	Third molar	(18–20 years)

Fractured teeth

In all instances where a tooth has been fractured or completely avulsed the possibility of inhalation of the tooth should be considered. If the missing tooth or fragment cannot be found then a chest X-ray should be considered to exclude an inhaled fragment. Inspiratory and expiratory views are required to look for obvious evidence of tooth fragments or for air trapping indicating obstruction to a lung segment. Inhaled teeth may present late as segmental collapse in association with infection.

Classification of tooth fractures

1. Fractures involving the enamel. These are not usually painful to hot and cold testing, routine referral to the GDP at the next available surgery for assessment is all that is required.

2. Fractures involving the enamel and dentine. Exposed dentine will be obvious as dentine is yellow, the tooth is exquisitely painful, sensitive to hot and cold testing and air. Referral to the general dental practitioner (GDP) for coating with a calcium hydroxide covering agent (e.g. Dycal) relieves pain and reduces the risk of infection.

3. Fractures involving the enamel, dentine and pulp. The pulp is visible as a red area in the fracture zone. Early referral for extirpation of the pulp is required to prevent abscess formation.

4. *Fractures involving the root.* Early referral is required for extirpation of the root.

Fractures involving the dentine, pulp or root should be referred to a dentist for treatment, covering the exposed area will reduce pain and minimize the risk of infection.

Displaced teeth

This injury is common in the primary teeth. The risk from such injuries is that the loose tooth may be inhaled. All such injuires should be referred to the dentist for extraction to prevent this complication. Reduction and splintage is not indicated.

Displaced permanent teeth should be preserved where possible for aesthetic reasons. Early intervention increases the probability that these teeth can survive. Definitive splinting of such teeth should be carried out by a dentist. In the absence of a dentist the tooth should be gently replaced in its socket under local anaesthesia and held in place for several minutes. If dental help is delayed a temporary spint may be made using aluminium foil (e.g. from the backing of a softgut suture packet). Simple analgesia and oral antibiotics should be prescribed (erythromycin or penicillin V 250–500 mg 6 hourly) and the patient referred to his or her GDP.

Avulsed teeth

Avulsed primary teeth should be discarded (or, since they have a certain commercial value, returned to their owner for appropriate disposal!).

Avulsed permanent teeth can be re-implanted; the prognosis is good if the tooth is handled correctly and re-implanted early. The temptation to discard an avulsed permanent tooth prior to dental assessment should be avoided as litigation could ensue as the prognosis from re-implantation is good.

1. *Initial management of the tooth.* The tooth should be cleaned in milk, the patient's own saliva or normal saline and gently placed back in the socket (alternately the tooth should be transported in milk or held in the buccal sulcus until dental help is obtained). The tooth should be splinted in place at the earliest opportunity by a dentist.

2. *Contraindications to re-implantation.*

- Primary teeth.
- History of rheumatic fever.
- Septal defects.
- Presence of prosthetic valves.
- Immunosuppressive therapy.
- Impaired conscious level (e.g. head injury).
- Compound fracture of maxilla or mandible.

Further reading

Hawksford J, Banks JG. *Maxillofacial and Dental Emergencies: Oxford Handbooks in Emergency Medicine.* Oxford: Oxford University Press, 1994.

Related topics of interest

Human and animal bites (p. 147)
Maxillofacial injuries (p. 195)
Ocular trauma (p. 212)

DIAPHRAGMATIC INJURIES

Diaphragmatic injuries are frequently difficult to diagnose and a high index of suspicion is required if they are not to be missed. Because they remain rare, few surgeons have extensive experience of their management.

Pathology

There is a predominance of left-sided lesions. This is due to the protective effect of the liver on the right side and possibly to the fact that the right hemidiaphragm is congenitally stronger than the left. Traumatic rupture of both sides of the diaphragm simultaneously has been reported.

Diaphragmatic rupture is associated with:

* High incidence of associated pelvic fractures in high-velocity trauma where massive forces produce dramatic changes in intra-abdominal pressure.
* High incidence of visceral injury in patients who have sustained blunt trauma.

Method of injury

The ratio of penetrating to blunt injury in diaphragmatic trauma is 2 : 1. Forces are transmitted to the diaphragm from the anterior abdominal wall or flank via the abdominal viscera. Knowledge of the mechanism of injury is vital in assessing the risk of injury to the diaphragm. This information is usually available from paramedics and other witnesses. Polaroid® photographs of vehicle wreckage may also be helpful if the patient has sustained injuries in a road-traffic accident. Other patients at risk include those who have fallen from a height, sustaining deceleration and crush injuries.

Diagnosis and investigation

1.   Penetrating trauma. Diagnosis of penetrating trauma is usually straightforward at laparotomy. However, small stab wounds can be missed and do not usually show herniation of a hollow viscus on plain radiography.

2.   Blunt trauma. Diagnosis in blunt trauma may be difficult, especially if herniation of abdominal organs has not occurred. Plain radiographs of patients with diaphragmatic rupture may be normal in up to 50% of cases, minor features which are suggestive and easily missed include:

* Obscuring of the diaphragmatic shadow.

- Apparent elevation of the diaphragm.

It is likely that laparoscopy and thoroscopy, which are usually effective, will have an increasing role to play in the diagnosis of diaphragmatic injuries. Ultrasonography may also be helpful. Peritoneal lavage may be negative.

Currently, the definitive method of confirming or excluding diaphragmatic rupture is exploratory laparotomy.

Treatment

The management of rupture of the diaphragm is surgical repair.

Further reading

Arak T, *et al.* Diaphragmatic injuries. *Injury,* 1997; **28:** 113–17.
Ochser MG, *et al.* Prospective evaluation of thoroscopy for diagnosis of diaphragmatic injury on thoraco-abdominal trauma. *Journal of Trauma,* 1993; **34:** 704.

Related topics of interest

ELBOW INJURIES: ADULTS

Elbow injuries are common, especially in children, and often present diagnostic and therapeutic problems. If incorrectly treated they can lead to serious long-term morbidity.

Fracture of the radial head

Mechanism of injury

These fractures usually occur as a result of falls on to an outstretched hand with a transmitted force along the forearm and a valgus deformity, therefore fracturing the radial head.

Clinical features

Clinical features include pain, swelling, restricted forearm pronation and supination, restricted elbow movements and tenderness over the head of the radius anteriorly and laterally (although the tenderness may be more diffuse).

Radiology

A positive fat pad sign is invariably present, although initially no other abnormality may be seen.

Management

Undisplaced fractures are initially treated symptomatically. Aspiration of the haemarthrosis and instillation of local anaesthetic may give considerable relief to patients in severe pain. Following initial rest, the elbow is mobilized in a collar and cuff with physiotherapy.

In rare cases with a single large fragment, open reduction and fixation may be appropriate, although the results can be disappointing.

In comminuted fractures, excision of the radial head is the treatment of choice. If this is undertaken in the acute phase, a short-term silastic spacer should be inserted to prevent radial shortening and consequent cubitus valgus deformity and its complications (including ulnar nerve palsy). The silastic spacer is removed after 6 months. When excision of the head is delayed and early movements encouraged there is invariably a persisting functional block, particularly to flexion, and late excision of the head and associated fragments and intra-articular debris will improve function.

Complications

Joint stiffness, particularly loss of extension and flexion.

Fracture of the radial neck

Mechanism of injury

Usually secondary to a fall on the outstretched hand. In the adult, fractures of the head of the radius are more common, in the child fractures of the neck.

Management

Minimally displaced fractures with angulation up to 20° are treated by early active movement following rest in a collar and cuff. Physiotherapy may be helpful. Significantly angulated fractures are treated by closed manipulation. Occasionally open reduction and stabilization with K-wires is necessary.

Fractures of the olecranon

Mechanism of injury

These injuries are usually due to a fall on to the elbow, striking the olecranon directly, resulting in some displacement. There is commonly an associated intra-articular component and damage to the articular surface.

Clinical features

Olecranon fractures are often compound due to the ease with which overlying tissues are damaged. Swelling, tenderness and bruising occur. Elbow extension may be limited or absent due to fragment displacement.

Radiology

Lateral radiography will confirm the fracture and demonstrate displacement.

Management

Compound fractures require debridement and consideration of early fixation. Undisplaced fractures can be managed with short-term plaster immobilization and observation to exclude displacement. Displaced fractures are treated by open reduction and fixation, usually using K-wires and a tension band.

Complications

- Pain and stiffness.
- Loss of function.
- Secondary osteoarthrosis (due to the presence of a residual articular step or other articular damage).
- Non-union (usually with reasonable function due to the formation of a fibrous union).

Fractures of the capitellum

Mechanism of injury   The usual mechanism of injury is a fall on an outstretched hand with the elbow straight, this fracture is more common in the elderly.

Clinical features   Pain, swelling, restricted movement and crepitus.

Radiology   Lateral radiography will demonstrate the proximal displacement of a significant component of the anterior surface of the capitellum and in some cases of the trochlear.

Management   Closed reduction is invariably unsuccessful as maintenance of the correct position is impossible. Open reduction is therefore the treatment of choice with fracture fixation using Herbert screws or excision of the bony fragment. Early mobilization produces the best functional result.

Dislocation of the elbow

Mechanism of injury   Dislocation of the elbow is usually an injury of adults although it occurs occasionally in children. The majority of dislocations are posterior (i.e. the distal component is displaced posteriorly) particularly postero-lateral. The injury usually results from a fall on an outstretched hand with the elbow extended.

Clinical features   The patient supports his arm, movement of which is exquisitely painful. Displacement is usually obvious. An assessment of neurovascular status is mandatory.

Radiology   Radiography confirms the nature and direction of the dislocation.

Management   The dislocation is reduced under anaesthesia. In view of the associated soft-tissue damage, the elbow is immobilized in plaster of Paris.

Complications
- Injury to the brachial artery (because the radial pulse may be present, this injury may not be immediately apparent).
- Compartment syndrome.
- Median or ulnar nerve injury (neuropraxia – spontaneous recovery is usual).

- Soft-tissue ossification and calcification with secondary loss of function. Myositis ossificans is a recognized complication and is particularly associated with excessive passive elbow mobilization. Resolution usually occurs with short-term splintage and anti-inflammatory medication. Rarely, late arthroscopy and capsulotomy may produce enhanced function.
- Re-dislocation due to gross disruption of associated ligament and capsular complexes. Regular follow-up is essential.

Further reading

Apley AG and Solomon L. *Apley's System of Orthopaedics and Fractures,* 7th Edn. Oxford: Butterworth Heinemann, 1993.

Related topics of interest

ELBOW INJURIES: CHILDREN

Supracondylar fractures

Mechanism of injury

Supracondylar fractures, although occurring occasionally in adults, are much more common in children. Most commonly there is posterior displacement of the distal fragment as a result of a fall on an outstretched hand.

Clinical features

The forearm is usually pronated and the proximal fragment may be prominent in the soft tissues anteriorly. Associated neurovascular injury may occur, most commonly to the brachial artery and median nerve (see below). Loss of passive finger extension may occur due to oedema in the flexor compartment caused by vascular compromise.

There is marked pain, tenderness and, in the case of displaced fractures, deformity.

Radiology

The fracture is confirmed by AP and lateral radiography.

Management

Early analgesia is mandatory. The arm should be assessed immediately for the presence of a neurovascular deficit: a pulseless arm in the presence of a supracondylar fracture is an orthopaedic emergency requiring immediate intervention. Closed reduction almost invariably restores the circulation. This is achieved by longitudinal traction with the forearm in the midprone position.

Where there is no displacement, the elbow is bent beyond 90° and immobilized in a collar and cuff. Alternatively, a temporary plaster back slab can be applied for comfort in the first few days. If flexion causes loss of pulses, the arm should be extended until they reappear: if this position does not maintain the reduction, immobilization in Dunlop traction may be necessary.

Displaced fractures require reduction under general anaesthesia. Following reduction the arm is immobilized as above. It is essential to ensure that the pulses are present following reduction, and if they are not, surgical exploration may be necessary.

Occasionally unstable fractures will require fixation with K-wires. Fractures that do not respond to closed manipulation may need open reduction and K-wire fixation.

Complications	• Vascular injury: usually to the brachial artery (see above).
	• Compartment syndrome: the median nerve and radial artery can be compressed by swelling in the anterior compartment of the forearm. Fasciotomy may be required. Paraesthesiae and pain on passive extension of the fingers is characteristic. The radial pulse may still be present in developing compartment syndrome.
	• Nerve damage: the median nerve usually remains intact and therefore recovery is usual.
	• Malunion: malunion is common unless a good position is achieved and may be unsightly. Loss of carrying angle or 'gunstock' deformity may occur. Corrective osteotomy may be necessary when growth is complete.
	• Volkman's ischaemic contracture.
	• Myositis ossificans.

Fracture of the medial epicondyle

Mechanism of injury	These injuries result from a varus stress caused by falls on to an outstretched hand with the wrist in extension. Avulsion occurs because of pull from the wrist flexors. Both this and lateral epicondylar injuries can be associated with joint dislocations, many of which will reduce spontaneously.
Clinical features	There is tenderness and swelling in relation to the medial epicondyle. Signs of ulnar nerve damage may be present.
Radiology	Standard radiographs will demonstrate the fracture, although comparison with a radiograph of the other, normal elbow may be necessary. The displaced epicondyle may be seen within the joint where it interferes with joint movement and may make an associated dislocation irreducible.
Treatment	Undisplaced fractures are managed conservatively with regular radiological observation. Displaced fractures must be reduced accurately, surgically if necessary, and fixed with K-wires.
Complications	• Ulnar nerve palsy.
	• Varus deformity due to growth arrest.
	• Pain and stiffness.

Fracture of the lateral epicondyle

Mechanism of injury   This fracture is most common in young children between the ages of 3 and 5 years and results from a fall and varus stress leading to an avulsion type fracture of the epiphysis.

Clinical features   The elbow is swollen and there is tenderness over the fracture site. Opposed wrist extension pulls on the lateral epicondyle, producing pain.

Radiology   Radiography confirms the bony avulsion. The fragment is invariably larger than the appearance on radiographs due to the presence of a cartilaginous component.

Management   Undisplaced fractures are treated in plaster with the elbow at 90° and the forearm pronated. As the injury is prone to slippage, regular radiography is necessary. Displaced fractures require accurate manipulation and fixation with K-wires. Open reduction is often required.

Complications
- Malunion: may result in residual deformity.
- Growth arrest: leading to residual deformity.
- Ulnar nerve palsy.

Pulled elbow

Mechanism of injury   This injury is especially common in young children and results from actions involving longitudinal traction to the arms, such as pulling a child to his feet or swinging a child by the arms. Subluxation of the orbicular ligament around the head of the radius occurs as the radial head is pulled out of it.

Clinical features   The child usually presents because a carer has noticed that he is not using his arm and cries when it is touched or moved. The arm may appear dangling and useless. Physical examination is usually unrewarding and a clinical diagnosis must be made based mainly on the mechanism of injury.

Radiology   In the presence of an appropriate history, radiography is unnecessary and should not be requested.

Management   The pulled elbow is reduced by swift pronation of the forearm with compression along the radius. The child cries, and normal function may return within minutes. A 'clunk' may be felt as the radial head returns to its normal position. If immediate recovery does not occur, the child should be reviewed after 1 hour, by which time the child will normally be using the arm. If no improvement has occurred, radiography should be requested to exclude a fracture. If the radiograph is normal and the child is still reluctant to use the arm, return of use will normally occur over a few days and appropriate follow-up should be arranged.

Pulled elbows often reduce spontaneously, frequently in the hospital waiting room or during (unnecessary) radiography.

Further reading

Apley AG and Solomon L. *Apley's System of Orthopaedics and Fractures,* 7th Edn. Oxford: Butterworth Heinemann, 1993.

Related topics of interest

Compartment syndrome (p. 70)
Injury patterns (p. 160)
Peripheral nerve injuries (p. 234)
Shoulder injuries (p. 265)
Vascular trauma (p. 317)

ENTONOX®

Entonox® is the trade name of a compressed gas mixture of 50% oxygen and 50% nitrous oxide.

Supply
- French blue cylinders with a white neck at a pressure of 137 bar (2000 lb/in^2 or 13 700 kPa).
- Premixed 50:50 nitrous oxide and oxygen delivered by pipeline at 4 bar (400 kPa).
- "Entonox" may be given from an anaesthetic machine using a resuscitation bag or anaesthetic circuit. This allows the proportions of oxygen and nitrous oxide to be varied and must be used with care as levels of deep anaesthesia may be achieved.

Physiology
- The two gases dissolve in each other at high pressures. The addition of oxygen to nitrous oxide lowers its critical temperature until at a 50:50 mixture it can be stored as a compressed gas. Under normal conditions there is no liquid in the cylinder.
- Cooling of a cylinder of Entonox® to a temperature below −7°C will cause separation of the two gases. This may result in the administration of, initially, an oxygen-rich mixture with inadequate analgesic properties and subsequently a hypoxic mixture, predominantly N_2O.
- Separation of Entonox® is more likely at a pressure of 117 bar (11 700 kPa) than at higher or lower pressures.
- When liquid nitrous oxide warms to its gaseous form, heat is taken from the bottle wall and frosting may result. The bottle should be kept remote from the patient if used in these circumstances.

Use

Entonox® cylinders in which separation is suspected should be gently inverted a few times before use, and all cylinders should be stored and used in the horizontal position.

Effects

1. *Rapid onset, rapid elimination.* This is due to relative insolubility of N_2O in blood. Once inhalation has occurred, the alveolar concentration falls rapidly, and the effect wears off after about 2 min.

2. *Non-cumulative.* There is no time limit to the use of Entonox®.

3. *Time lag.* This is approximately 1 min before an analgesic effect is achieved.

4. *Administration.* Given (conventionally) by patient activated demand valve. Appropriate instructions to the patient are required. The demand valve can be overridden by medical staff, but drowsiness and deep anaesthesia may result.

5. *Confidence.* Inadequate 'predosage' will result in loss of patient confidence.

Contraindications

1. *'The Bends' – Caisson disease.* An absolute contraindication as nitrous oxide diffuses rapidly into air filled spaces such as air emboli, the pleural cavity, bowel, middle ear and cranial cavity.

2. *Pneumothorax.* Entonox® is absolutely contraindicated in established pneumothorax and relatively contraindicated in patients at risk of pneumothorax due to the presence of significant chest injuries (unless chest drains have been placed).

3. *Head injuries.* This is controversial but its use is probably acceptable if associated (non-cranial) injuries are painful and require analgesia.

4. *Patients requiring high flow oxygen.* Entonox® is only 50% oxygen, patients requiring high flow oxygen should receive O_2 via a rebreathing (Hudson) mask and intravenous or regional anaesthesia.

5. *Facial injuries.* Practical considerations prevent the use of Entonox® in such patients.

Indications

- As a supplement to intravenous analgesia in reduction of shoulder dislocations.
- As a supplement in incomplete nerve blocks.
- For the application of splints.
- In isolated limb fractures.
- For the reduction of dislocated fingers or patellae.

The following side-effects may be noted:

- Confusion.
- Restlessness.

- Dizziness.
- Drowsiness.

Further reading

Aitkenhead AR, Smith G (eds). *Textbook of Anaesthetics*, 2nd Edn. Edinburgh: Churchill Livingstone, 1990.
Craft TM, Upton PM (eds). *Key Topics in Anaesthesia*, 2nd Edn. Oxford: BIOS Scientific Publishers, 1995.

Related topics of interest

FAT EMBOLISM SYNDROME

Fat embolism was first demonstrated histologically by Zanker in 1862; however, despite this early recognition, controversy still exists regarding its aetiology. Although associated with long bone fractures, fat embolism syndrome has been recorded following soft-tissue injuries, burns and some non-traumatic conditions. Fat embolism occurs following trauma-related procedures and elective arthroplasty. It probably occurs in the majority of long bone fractures and pelvic fractures, yet most patients remain asymptomatic or will develop subclinical mild hypoxia. The fully established syndrome is associated with a mortality of 10–15%.

Incidence

Unless specifically sought, mild cases of fat embolism may not be recognized as they may only be demonstrated on blood gas analysis. Szabo *et al.* (1963) demonstrated 100% consistency of evidence of the presence of fat embolism in a large series of patients suffering fatalities due to major trauma. Peltier (1969) reported an incidence of fat embolism in 3.4% of tibial fractures, 9% of femoral fractures and 20% of patients with combined tibial and femoral fractures.

Pathology and aetiology

There are two theories of aetiology: the mechanical theory and the metabolic theory:

- The mechanical theory suggests that bone marrow enters the bloodstream through torn-open venous channels. However, as stated above, fat embolism can occur in the absence of trauma and certainly in the absence of long bone fractures. Furthermore, it has been demonstrated by transoesophageal ultrasonography that showers of emboli occur during intramedullary nailing without producing clinical signs or symptoms.
- The metabolic theory postulates an alternative aetiology, and suggests that circulating chylomicrons aggregate as a secondary effect of trauma. Possible initiating factors include the release of lipase from damaged tissues. It is suggested that the clinical manifestations begin with the release of free fatty acids by pulmonary lipase or lipase released by the injured tissues, which in turn initiate the inflammatory and clotting cascades and the complement system. Tissue damage is increased by oxygen free-radicals and activated proteases. As a result of this, capillary leakage occurs, with local oedema and haemorrhage,

alveolar collapse and consequent ventilation–perfusion mismatch leading to hypoxia.

Clinical features

Symptoms and signs of fat embolism usually manifest themselves between 12 and 72 hours following injury:

- Otherwise unexplained pyrexia occurring too soon to be likely to be due to an infective process (usually 12–24 hours after injury).
- Altered level of consciousness due to cerebral oedema and microinfarction.
- Tachycardia.
- Raised (or normal) respiratory rate.
- Hypoxia is invariable and the pO_2 is usually in the region of 8 kPa.
- Hypercapnia.
- Skin petechiae on the trunk and limbs (and occasionally the conjunctivae or oral mucosa). More than six are regarded as diagnostic.

Routine analysis of blood gases following major long bone fractures in the absence of associated chest injuries or any clinical evidence of fat embolism syndrome shows deranged gases in up to one-third of patients. It has been suggested that when contemplating intramedullary nailing, there is an increased risk of fulminating fat embolism syndrome if hypoxia is apparent on pre-operative blood gas analysis. Furthermore, the likelihood of fat embolism syndrome following intramedullary nailing is suggested by intra-operative pyrexia.

Pulse oximetry, while giving reassurance regarding oxygen saturation, can, in the presence of supplemental oxygen, mask the alveolar hypoventilation and hypercapnia seen in fat embolism syndrome.

Confusion and changes in mental state are more common than focal neurological deficit. In the head-injured patient, the onset of confusion is an indication for cranial CT scanning in order to exclude any intracerebral pathology due directly to trauma.

Investigation

- Radiographic changes characterized by multiple diffuse pulmonary infiltrates usually occur some time after initial clinical suspicions.
- Arterial blood gas estimation should be routine after long bone fracture and the diagnostic pO_2 will be less than 8 kPa.

- Thombocytopenia may occur, with platelet counts being less than 150 000/mm^3. The main consumption of platelets is in pulmonary aggregates.
- Clotting abnormalities vary from mild to disseminated intravascular coagulation.
- Fat may be demonstrated in sputum and urine. This may occur in the trauma victim in the absence of fat embolism syndrome.

Treatment

Treatment is largely supportive, with high-flow oxygen therapy and ventilation if the pO_2 can not be maintained above 8 kPa. Positive end-expiratory pressure (PEEP) is of value in reopening collapsed alveoli. Monitoring should include regular blood gas analysis, chest X-ray, blood and platelet counts. The patient's neurological state should be reviewed regularly. Neither heparin nor corticosteroids have been proven to be of any benefit.

Prevention

Early fracture stabilization may be achieved manually with simple longitudinal traction and converted to appropriate splintage on the arrival of the emergency services. Unrecognized hypoxia and hypovolaemia are probably the most important precipitating factors of fat embolism and may be avoided by careful resuscitation. It has been suggested that early fracture fixation reduces the incidence of fat embolism, although this remains controversial.

Further reading

Metcalf S. Fat embolism syndrome. Greaves I, Porter K, Ryan J (eds) In: *Trauma 1*. London: Arnold, 1997.

Peltier LF. Fat embolism – a current concept. *Clinical Orthopaedics and Related Research,* 1969; **66:** 241–53.

Szabo G, Serenyi P, Kocsar L. Fat embolism: fat absorption from the site of injury. *Surgery,* 1963; **54:** 756–60.

Related topics of interest

FOOT FRACTURES: MID AND FOREFOOT

Mid-tarsal and tarso-metatarsal injuries

These injuries result from equinus forces, for example in road-traffic accident foot pedal injuries. The degree of injury varies from simple ligamentous strain through simple fractures to fracture dislocation. These injuries may be complicated by compartment syndrome.

Presentation

The foot is bruised and swollen, associated loss of function depends on the severity of the injury.

Investigation

It is easy to miss fractures on plain radiographs, particularly if spontaneous relocation has occurred. Metatarsal bone fragments should raise the possibility of previous dislocation. CT scanning may be necessary for the assessment of patients requiring operative intervention.

Treatment

1. *Undisplaced fractures.* Minor fractures with minimal symptoms can be treated with rest, ice, compression and elevation (RICE). Immobilization in plaster for 4–6 weeks may be necessary.

2. *Displaced fractures.* Open reduction and internal fixation should be considered.

3. *Fracture dislocations.* Following CT assessment, closed manipulation or open reduction with K wire fixation in both cases is appropriate.

The classical *Lisfranc dislocation* involves a diastasis between the first and second metatarsals. The most important prognostic factor is loss of the longitudinal arch of the foot, which requires surgical intervention. When the arch is preserved and displacement minimal, conservative treatment produces good results.

Complications

Compartment syndrome may occur early, initial suspicion is clinical with confirmation by pressure studies. Surgical decompression is required. Secondary osteoarthrosis may occur.

Metatarsal injuries

The mechanisms of injury are:

- Direct trauma (for example, crush from a falling heavy object).
- Twisting injuries.
- Repetitive stress ('march fracture', usually of the second metatarsal).

Presentation

The foot is diffusely swollen across the dorsum, with tenderness and bruising. Fractures of the base of the fifth metatarsal demonstrate tenderness over the proximal part of the lateral aspect of the foot. Such fractures are often associated with avulsions from inversion injuries of the ankle.

Treatment

1. *Shaft fractures.* Crush injuries require rest, ice and elevation with immobilization in a light support (double tubigrip) or walking plaster. Marked displacement is treated by closed manipulation (and, if necessary, open reduction and K wiring, especially if the first or fifth metatarsals are fractured).

2. *Fractures of the base of the fifth metatarsal.* Undisplaced fractures of the base of the fifth metatarsal associated with inversion injuries are treated in a light support or a weight-bearing plaster for approximately 6 weeks, depending on the degree of symptoms. Some non-articular fractures of the base of the fifth metatarsal may require open reduction and internal fixation.

3. *March fractures.* Support in a double tubigrip for 2–3 weeks is usually all that is required. If the pain is severe, a below-knee walking plaster may be appropriate. Recurrence can be prevented by the provision of a suitable orthotic shoe insert. Initial radiographs may be normal, the fracture only becoming apparent with the development of callous on subsequent films. Nuclear bone scanning will provide an immediate diagnosis.

Metatarso-phalangeal injuries

These range from sprains to fracture dislocations, occurring most commonly in athletes. Dislocations are reduced and protected in a light, weight-bearing cast for 4 weeks. Sprains are treated symptomatically.

Phalangeal fractures

Fractures are usually the result of a weight falling on to the toes or, usually in the case of the fifth toe, due to abduction strain from the foot striking a stationary object.

Treatment is symptomatic with pain relief, elevation and compression strapping. If there is no evidence of displacement or compound injury, radiography is not usually required. Occasionally, closed manipulation of angulated fractures is required.

Sesamoid fractures

Sesamoid fractures are usually due to the impact of a heavy object landing on the toe, and most commonly affect the medial sesamoid. Most settle spontaneously with conservative treatment. Occasionally, plaster immobilization is required for symptomatic relief. Subsequent physiotherapy may be necessary. If discomfort persists, injection of local anaesthetic and steroids or surgical excision may be required.

Further reading

McRae R. *Practical Fracture Treatment*, 3rd Edn. Edinburgh: Churchill Livingstone, 1994.

Related topics of interest

Ankle injuries: fractures (p. 30)
Ankle injuries: sprains (p. 34)
Compartment syndrome (p. 70)
Foot fractures: talus and calcaneum (p. 99)
Sports injuries (p. 280)

FOOT FRACTURES: TALUS AND CALCANEUM

Fractures of the bones of the feet are common, often badly managed and frequently missed. Inadequate treatment of these fractures may lead to long-term problems and disability.

Talar fractures

Talar fractures are rare and are usually associated with high-velocity trauma in road-traffic accidents. These fractures were recognized by Anderson in 1919 and termed 'aviator's astragalus'.

Anatomy

- Fractures can involve the body, neck, head or lateral process of the talus.
- Subtalar, talonavicular and total talar dislocations may occur.
- Blood supply is via the anterior tibial, posterior tibial and peroneal vessels. Intraosseous blood supply runs in an antero-posterior direction.
- Fractures of the neck of the talus are particularly prone to vascular complications and are classified according to the Hawkins classification:

  Type 1. Minimal displacement or no displacement: only one source of blood supply compromised.

  Type 2. Subtalar subluxation or dislocation: at least two sources of blood supply compromised.

  Type 3 . Body of talus dislocated: all sources of blood supply compromised with a high risk of avascular necrosis.

Treatment

The principles of management of talar fractures are as follows:

- Early reduction of dislocations and fracture dislocations should be carried out to prevent skin necrosis.
- Compound fractures require surgical debridement and delayed primary closure or skin grafting.
- Undisplaced talar neck fractures are treated in plaster of Paris, with the foot plantigrade for 8 weeks. The plaster is not weight bearing in fractures of the neck and body, but weight bearing in fractures of the head.
- Displaced fractures and fracture dislocations of the neck of the talus may be treated by closed

manipulation, but often open reduction and fixation (usually with lag screws) are required. Patients treated conservatively require immobilization in plantar flexion in plaster for 2–3 weeks, followed by 6–8 weeks in a neutral position.

- Displaced fractures of the body, head or lateral processes are treated in a similar way. Large bony fragments require open reduction and fixation.

Fractures of the body and head of the talus usually have a good prognosis unless associated with gross soft-tissue injury. Fractures of the neck of talus, because of associated vascular compromise, often produce a poor outcome.

Complications

1. *Skin damage.* May be prevented by early reduction.

2. *Avascular necrosis.* Occurs in approximately 50% of talar neck fractures. Many cases will settle eventually, with reasonable function if protected from weight bearing.

3. *Malunion.* Malunion producing pain, especially on weight bearing, is a predisposing factor for secondary osteoarthrosis.

4. *Secondary osteoarthrosis.* Malunion, avascular necrosis and the degree of initial trauma all contribute to the development of secondary osteoarthrosis.

Calcaneal fractures

Calcaneal fractures account for 60% of tarsal bone fractures and 2% of all fractures. Most are intra-articular, affecting the subtalar joint.

Mechanism of injury

Talar fractures are usually associated with falls from a height, landing on the heels. The fracture is produced as the calcaneus is driven upwards against the talus. In these patients, it is important to exclude hip and spine fractures resulting from the same mechanism.

Occasionally avulsion fractures may occur (e.g. at the insertion of the achilles tendon) or fractures may result from direct trauma.

Clinical features

Pain and inability to weight bear are common, although they may be absent. Bruising develops on the sole of the foot and the heel appears broadened if viewed from behind.

Classification

Primary and secondary fracture lines generated when the talus cleaves the calcaneus from above can be recognized on plain radiographs. The primary fracture line crosses the posterior facet of the subtalar joint, separating a medial sustenacular fragment from a large inferolateral fragment. The fracture line then continues over the posterior articular facet and the body, from postero-medial to antero-lateral.

Commonly, a secondary fracture line divides the inferolateral part of the bone into a lateral joint fragment (thalamic fragment) and a body fragment, thus producing a three-part fracture.

Essex-Lopresti classified the three-part fractures into two groups, based on the appearance of the fracture line seen on the lateral radiographs:

- 'Tongue' type, involving a fracture running posteriorly through the body to reach the posterior aspect below the insertion of the Achilles tendon.
- 'Joint depression fragment', where the secondary fracture line passes down to the lateral side of the calcaneum behind the posterior articular facet.

Eastwood *et al.* have produced a fracture classification which is a mandatory part of the assessment of any patient requiring operative intervention and is based on the appearance of the lateral wall on coronal CT scanning:

- *Type 1*, the lateral wall is formed solely by the lateral joint fragment.
- *Type 2*, the lateral wall is formed by the lateral joint fragment superiorly and the body fragment inferiorly.
- *Type 3*, the lateral wall is formed solely by the body fragment.

Treatment

Initial treatment involves hospital admission for leg elevation and analgesia as well as the application of ice until the swelling subsides. During this period, necessary investigations can be undertaken. Plain radiographs including lateral oblique and axial films, should be obtained. Evidence of the displacement of the fracture is determined by measuring Böhler's angle (*Figure 1*).

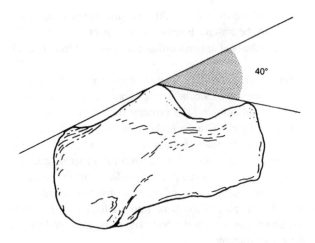

Figure 1. Böhler's angle. Reproduced from Burke, Greaves and Hormbrey (1996) *Self Assessment in Accident and Emergency Medicine* with permission from Butterworth Heinemann.

1. Extra-articular fractures. These fractures are treated with rest and ice then non-weight-bearing plaster and crutches for 6 weeks.

2. Displaced avulsions. Reduction and fixation is carried out, followed by 4–6 weeks immobilization in a weight-bearing plaster.

3. Intra-articular fractures. Undisplaced or minimally displaced intra-articular fractures are treated as extra-articular fractures.

Displaced intra-articular fractures are treated by open reduction and internal fixation (with bone grafting where required), followed by a non-weight-bearing plaster for 8 weeks. Recovery in displaced fractures is slow and generally unsatisfactory if conservative treatment is attempted, due to joint disruption and malunion.

Accurate reduction, stable fixation and early joint mobilization constitute sound objectives for the management of these fractures.

Complications

The following complications may occur:

- Skin blistering.
- Malunion (usually valgus, with a broad heel).
- Peroneal tendon infringement due to the valgus heel.

- Fibular abutment (the fibula catches on the side of the calcaneum).
- Stiffness and secondary osteoarthrosis.

For treatment of significant secondary osteoarthrosis with pain and stiffness, subtalar arthrodesis produces the most satisfactory results.

Further reading

Eastwood DM *et al.* Intra-articular fractures of the calcaneum. *Journal of Bone and Joint Surgery,* 1995; **75B** (2): 183–8.
Essex-Lopresti P. The mechanism, reduction techniques and results in fractures of the os calcis. *British Journal of Surgery,* 1952; **39:** 395–419.

Related topics of interest

GENITOURINARY TRAUMA

Genitourinary trauma presents a challenge to the trauma team. The kidneys, ureters and bladder are hidden by the retroperitoneal space and pelvis, and are therefore not amenable to standard clinical examination. Clinical signs of genitourinary trauma may be subtle or absent in the early stages or may be masked by the presence of other injuries.

Penetrating genitourinary trauma is uncommon in the UK and accounts for approximately 5% of all cases. Most cases are associated with injuries to other intra-abdominal or retro-peritoneal structures.

Upper urinary tract

History

In the majority of cases a history of direct blunt trauma to the abdomen or flank is elicited. Such injuries result in crushing of the kidney between the externally applied force and either the lumbar spine, 12th rib or paravertebral muscles. In a few cases a history of decelerating injury, such as a fall from a height, should suggest the possibility of indirect renal trauma. Such injuries cause tearing of the major vessels at the renal pedicle, or avulsion of the ureter at the pelviureteric junction. A history of frank haematuria should be sought, although the absence of frank haematuria does not exclude significant injury. (In avulsion injuries of the renal pedicle 70% of cases have no evidence of frank haematuria due to disruption of the blood supply to the kidney.)

Examination

The clinical signs of renal trauma include:
- Flattening of the normal loin contour and loin mass due to a perinephric haematoma.
- Local abrasions or bruising in the flank.
- Local bruising or imprinting on the anterior abdominal wall.
- Tenderness over the loin.
- Entry or exit wounds (in penetrating trauma).
- Frank haematuria (in significant renal trauma).
- Paralytic ileus (due to a perinephric haematoma).
- Hypovolaemic shock.

Classification of renal trauma (based upon clinical and radiological findings)

1. Minor (85%). Contusions or superficial lacerations in which the capsule and pelvicalyceal system is intact.

2. *Major (10%)*. Deep lacerations with involvement of the capsule and/or the pelvi-calyceal system.

3. *Critical (5%)*. Injuries involving the pedicle with avulsion of vessels and disruption of the pelvi-ureteric junction.

Investigations

Intravenous urography is the investigation of choice in most cases of suspected upper urinary tract trauma. Indications for intravenous urogram (IVU) include:

- Frank haematuria.
- Microscopic haematuria in the presence of shock.
- Prior to laparotomy if renal trauma is suspected to confirm the presence of renal tract trauma and to confirm the presence of a functional kidney.

Renal ultrasound may be used in haemodynamically stable patients suspected of having renal trauma, and to image kidneys which do not show up on IVU. Computed tomography (CT) scanning with contrast provides no more information than the two previous investigations.

Management

The majority of cases of renal trauma (95%) can be managed conservatively. Indications for surgery include patients with critical injuries and those with major injuries who are haemodynamically unstable.

Patients with microscopic haematuria persisting for more than 1 week warrant further investigation.

Lower urinary tract

The basic principle in managing a patient with a suspected lower urinary tract injury is not to pass a urinary catheter without first considering and excluding the possibility of a urethral injury. If a urethral injury is suspected then a urological opinion should be obtained prior to catheterization.

Bladder

Bladder injuries are uncommon. They are caused by direct trauma to a distended bladder, or by penetration of the bladder by a bony fragment from a pelvic fracture. The diagnosis is often delayed because the injury is not suspected, or the patient may be intoxicated or suffering from a head injury. Failure to pass urine should suggest the injury in such cases. Lower abdominal peritonism may be present, but may be attributed to intra-abdominal pathology.

Investigations	The standard pelvic film requested on all major trauma victims may show a pelvic fracture, which should alert the diagnostician to the possibility of bladder perforation. A diastasis of the symphysis pubis suggests the possibility of a urethral injury.
	Contract studies will confirm the diagnosis. Either IVU or cystography can be performed. IVU is done first if upper renal tract trauma is suspected. Cystography is performed if bladder trauma alone is suspected and a urinary catheter is in place.
Treatment	Intraperitoneal injuries require surgical repair and suprapubic and urethral bladder drainage. Extraperitoneal injuries require urethral drainage only.
Urethral injuries	Urethral injuries are rare in women. Bulbar injuries present with a classical history of a fall astride a hard object. Membranous urethral injuries are usually secondary to a pelvic fracture or diastasis of the symphysis. Perineal bruising, blood at the urethral meatus and difficulty or inability to pass urine are common findings. In addition injuries to the membranous urethra are associated with pelvic fracture and high riding prostate. All patients with suspected urethral injury should have early urological assessment prior to any attempt to pass a urinary catheter. In patients who cannot pass urine a suprapubic catheter is placed and elective urethorgraphy is performed to determine the site and degree of injury. In the presence of a high riding prostate an IVU may be required to exclude disruption and displacement of the bladder.
	Gentle urethral catheterization may be attempted in the presence of a pelvic fracture if the following conditions are met:

- The symphysis pubis is intact.
- There is no blood at the tip of the urethra.
- There is no perineal bruising.

Further reading

American College of Surgeons Committee on Trauma. Abdominal trauma. In: *Advanced Trauma Life Support: Program for Physicians.* Chicago: American College of Surgeons, 1993; 141–58.

Blandy J. *Lecture Notes on Urology*, 4th Edn. Oxford: Blackwell Scientific Publications, 1989.

Skinner D, Driscoll P, Earlam R. *ABC of Major Trauma*. London: BMJ Publications, 1991; 46–50.

Related topics of interest

GLASGOW COMA SCORE

The Glasgow Coma *Score* is a derivative of the Glasgow Coma *Scale*, first described by Teasdale and Jennett in 1974. They described a clinical scale consisting of assessment of eye, verbal, and motor responses to defined stimuli. The authors specified that normal flexion (rapid withdrawal associated with abduction of the shoulder) and abnormal flexion (slower, stereotyped assumption of the hemiplegic or decorticate posture with adduction of the shoulder) should be included under the same heading of flexion, as inexperienced observers might find it difficult to differentiate between the two. Each modality of response was recorded separately on a graph, no attempt being made to integrate the individual modalities to produce a global description of conscious level, or to assign a numerical score.

Modalities

Motor responses

1. Obeying commands. The terms 'purposeful' and 'voluntary' are avoided as there is no objective definition of the terms. Grasp reflexes or postural adjustments in response to verbal stimuli are excluded.

In the absence of a response to a specific command, a painful stimulus is applied. This requires a standardized stimulus maintained until the maximal response is obtained. Initially pressure is applied to the nailbed with a pencil which may elicit either flexion or extension at the elbow. If flexion is observed, the painful stimulus is applied to the head, neck and trunk to test for localization. A spinal reflex may still be present in the lower limbs with brainstem death, causing flexion in response to locally applied pain. The painful stimulus is therefore best applied to the upper limbs.

2. Localizing response. Painful stimulus at more than one site results in movement of a limb to remove the stimulus.

3. Flexor response. Normal or abnormal flexion in response to a painful stimulus.

4. Extensor posturing. Adduction and internal rotation of the forearm and pronation of the forearm in response to a painful stimulus. The term 'decerebrate rigidity', is avoided as it suggests a specific physio-anatomical correlation.

5. No response. To adequate deep pain stimulus, in the absence of cord transection.

The best response correlates with the functional state of the brain, differential responses in different limbs suggest focal brain injury. Both the best and worse response and the location of each response should be recorded.

Verbal responses

1. Orientation. Awareness of self and the environment. The individual should know who (s)he is, where (s)he is and why (s)he is there. In addition patients should know the year, season and month. The terms 'rational' and 'sensible' are excluded from the definition as having no objective meaning.

2. Confused conversation. Attention can be held and the patient responds to questions in a conversational manner, but the responses indicate disorientation and confusion.

3. Inappropriate speech. Intelligent articulation used only in an exclamatory or random manner, usually in the form of swearing or shouting. Conversational speech is not possible.

4. Incomprehensible speech. Moaning and groaning without any recognizable words.

5. No response. The stimulus required to elicit a confused, incomprehensible or no verbal response was not defined in the original paper, but is generally taken to be either a verbal or painful stimulus (usually nailbed pressure with a pencil).

Eye opening

1. Spontaneously. Indicates that brainstem arousal mechanisms are functional, but does not imply awareness.

2. To speech. Eye opening to any verbal stimulus whether spoken or shouted. This does not have to be a specific command to open the eyes.

3. To pain. This is tested by application of a painful stimulus to a limb. Application of painful stimuli to the supraorbital ridge or angle of the jaw may result in eye closure due to reflex grimacing.

4. *No response.*

The Glasgow Coma Scale has been adopted worldwide as the standard method of assessing conscious level.

The Glasgow Coma Score

This is basically the Glasgow Coma Scale with the inclusion of abnormal flexion as a separate category of motor response to pain. In addition, numerical scoring of the responses in each modality has been introduced along with a summary numerical score which is the total of the three individual modality scores. The Glasgow Coma Score forms part of the ATLS Secondary Survey.

The Glasgow Coma Score

Eye response (range 1–4)		Verbal response (range 1–5)		Motor response (range 1–6)	
Opens spontaneously	4	Orientated	5	Obeys commands	6
To speech	3	Confused	4	To pain	
To pain	2	Inappropriate	3	Localizes	5
None	1	Incomprehensible	2	Normal flexion	4
		None	1	Abnormal flexion	3
				Extension	2
				None	1

Total GCS = Eye score +Motor score + Verbal score

The Glasgow Coma Score is a component of many physiological scoring systems (e.g. Revised Trauma Score, APACHE III) either as the actual score, or as a weighted score based upon subgroups of the total score.

It should always be remembered that the true value of the Glasgow Coma Score lies in the observation of trends over a period of time rather than in any one value.

Children's Coma Score

The verbal component of the Glasgow Coma Score is not appropriate to younger children. For this reason several modified scales have been introduced. The scale given below is one of the more commonly used and has the advantage that it covers the same numerical range as the Glasgow Coma Score. It is recommended for use in children under the age of 4 years.

Children's Coma Score

Eye response (range 1–4)		Motor response (range 1–5)		Verbal response (range 1–5)		
Opens spontaneously	4	Spontaneously obeys commands	6	Smiles, orientated to sounds, follows objects, interacts		5
To speech	3	To pain				
To pain	2	Localizes	5	*If crying*	*If interacts*	
None	1	Withdraws	4	Consolable	Inappropriately	4
		Abnormal flexion (decorticate)	3	Inconsistently consolable	Moaning	3
		Extension (decerebrate)				
		None	2	Inconsolable	Irritable	2
			1	No response	No response	1

Although the validity of the Glasgow Coma Score is well established, the validity of the Children's Coma Score is not. Several other systems have been proposed, some of which are in the process of validation.

Further reading

Glasgow JFT, Graham H. *Management of Injuries in Children.* London: BMJ Publishing Group, 1997.
Teasdale G, Jennett B. Assessment of coma and impaired consciousness. *Lancet,* 1974; 81–4.

Related topics of interest

Brainstem death and organ transplantation (p. 50)
Head injuries (p. 124)
Paediatric aspects of trauma (p. 216)

GUNSHOT INJURIES

Although still rare in the UK, gunshot wounds are becoming more common as crime, particularly drug related crime, becomes more violent.

Physiology

- The damage done to tissue by a missile depends on the amount of energy given up to that tissue by the missile.
- The potential energy for tissue damage is given by the formula:

$$E = \frac{MV^2}{2}$$

where M is the mass of the bullet and V its velocity.

- A tenfold increase in the bullet's mass increases its energy tenfold, a tenfold increase in its velocity increases its energy 100 fold.
- If a bullet is stopped by tissue, the energy liberated is equal to the kinetic energy, if the bullet passes through a body the energy liberated is proportional to the difference between the entry and exit velocities.
- Tissue damage depends on:

1. *Factors relating to the missile.*

- Velocity.
- Mass.
- Shape.
- Size.
- Stability.
- Composition.

2. *Factors relating to the tissues.*

- Composition.
- Density.
- Elasticity.

All these factors effect missile retardation. The more rapid the retardation the greater the energy release and tissue damage.

Yaw, precession and nutation

Bullets are aerodynamically unstable and whilst in the air are subject to:
- Yaw (tumbling).
- Precession and nutation (spinning due to rifling of the gun barrel).

Travelling in the air these effects are stabilized due to the gyroscopic action of spin, this does not happen as effectively in tissues denser than air thus causing instability, tumbling and tissue destruction (*Figure 1*).

(a)

(b)

(c)

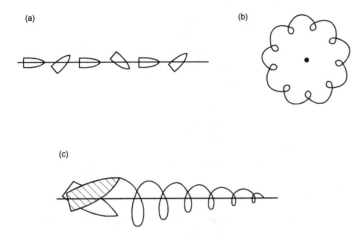

Figure 1. (a) Yaw, (b) precession and (c) nutation.

Although a stable perforating bullet may use up less than 20% of its available energy, an unstable bullet will give up a greater proportion, causing much greater tissue damage. Irregularly shaped missiles (such as bomb fragments) are much less stable than regular ones and are associated with significant tissue damage.

Types of bullet

- Full metal jacketed: under the Hague Convention military ammunition must have a complete metal covering to prevent deformation on impact.
- Civilian and police ammunition: this is not surrounded by a metal jacket and is designed to deform on impact producing maximum tissue damage. This is to prevent collateral damage by bullets passing through their intended victim and to increase the chance of an instant kill or disablement when dealing, for example, with terrorists.

Fragmentation

- Fragmentation increases tissue destruction and is proportional to the thickness of the metal jacket and to the velocity and inversely proportional to the range.
- Some ammunition is designed with a weakness (or cannelure) in the metal jacket so that the bullet breaks at that point. (*Figure 2*).

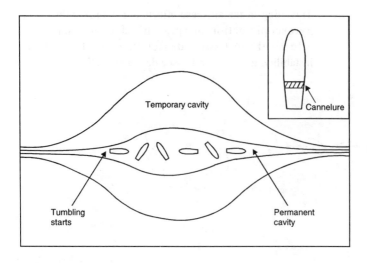

Figure 2. Wound profile – high velocity (inset: cannelured round).

Missile path

Missiles are diverted by resistance from tissues of different densities. It is impossible to predict the path of a high velocity bullet from its entrance point.

Tissue damage

Bullets produce tissue damage in three ways

1.   Laceration and crushing. This is due to the direct effect of the missile passing through the tissue. This is the main effect of low velocity weapons with bullets travelling at less than 350 m/sec (the velocity of sound in air). Bullets from the majority of hand guns and submachine guns are of this type.

2.   Shock wave. A shock wave travelling at 1500 m/sec is produced by compression of tissue in front of the penetrating missile. This produces short duration pressure changes of up to 100 atmospheres.

3.   Temporary cavitation. Produced by high velocity missiles, the energy of the bullet is transmitted to the tissues causing them to expand away from it and producing a temporary cavity 30–40 times the diameter of the bullet. The sub-atmospheric pressure within the cavity sucks in debris and bacteria thus contaminating lacerated tissue planes. The temporary cavity then collapses to leave a smaller permanent cavity.

Effects on different tissues

Temporary cavitation has different effects on different tissues:

- Soft tissues are destroyed.
- Small vessels are disrupted.
- Larger vessels and nerves are stretched.
- Bone may be shattered (producing secondary missiles).

Direct bone strike necessarily results in high energy transfer. In general, solid organs such as liver, brain and muscle are more susceptible than air containing organs such as lung and bowel.

Management

1. *First priority*. Resuscitation with ABC.

2. *Second priority*. Mainly surgical with tissue repair and prevention of infective complications:
- All gunshot wounds should be assumed to be heavily contaminated with bacteria, particular dangers being *Clostridium tetani* and *C. perfringens* (gas gangrene).
- In general all gunshot wounds (with the possible exception of isolated through and through chest wounds) should undergo surgical exploration and wound toilet.
- Following surgical debridement wounds are left open with delayed primary closure after 4 or 5 days.

Further reading

Blast and gunshot injury. In Greaves I, Dyer P, Porter K (eds). *A Handbook of Immediate Care*. London: W B Saunders, 1995.
Kirby NG, Blackburn G (eds). *Field Surgery Pocket Book*. London: HMSO, 1981.
Ryan J, Cooper G (eds). *Ballistic Trauma*. London: Arnold, 1997.

Related topics of interest

Amputation: traumatic (p. 18)
Penetrating cardiac injury (p. 229)
Psychological aspects of trauma (p. 249)
Tetanus and gas gangrene (p. 286)

HAND INJURIES

Hand injuries comprise approximately 10% of all 'minor injuries' presenting to the A&E Department. Although apparently trivial, if treated inadequately such injuries may lead to significant loss of function and consequent morbidity. Such inadequately treated injuries are a common cause for complaint and frequently attract the attention of solicitors.

Metacarpal fractures

Fractures of the shaft or neck of a metacarpal rarely cause problems. The most common mechanism of injury is from fights in which the clenched fist strikes a hard object.

'Boxer's fracture'	Fractures of the neck of the fifth metacarpal ('boxer's fracture') do not normally require reduction, indeed it is difficult to do a closed reduction of such fractures, and maintaining such reduction may be difficult. Very occasionally, for example in the young, or those requiring exceptional hand function (for example pianists), operative intervention may be required.The main complication of conservative management of such fractures is loss of the normal contour of the knuckle, this leads to little functional impairment. Early mobilization by neighbour strapping to the fourth digit for 7–10 days reduces the incidence and degree of extensor lag associated with this injury.
Spiral fractures	Spiral fractures of the shaft rarely lead to any significant functional loss if treated conservatively. Such injuries may be missed if only AP views are requested: lateral and/or oblique views should be obtained.
	Spiral fractures of the metacarpals without angulation, and multiple fractures of the metacarpals are best managed in a volar slab, with the metacarpophalangeal joints flexed to 90° and the interphalangeal joints extended to 180° (the position of function) for 7–10 days.
Fractures with deformity	Occasionally a fracture of a metacarpal may result in significant angulation and rotational deformity (demonstrated by asking the patient to clench their fist): internal fixation is often required to hold such injuries in correct alignment.

Phalangeal fractures

Single fractures of the proximal phalanx may be either transverse or oblique and both may give rise to problems when managed conservatively.

Transverse fractures are prone to angulation. If relatively undisplaced, they may be managed in a volar slab. During the first 10 days they are prone to displacement and angulation and frequent follow-up during this time is required. Failure to maintain position is an indication for open reduction and internal fixation.

Spiral fractures are prone to rotational deformity which, if untreated, will lead to crossing over of the finger tips when a fist is made. Fractures associated with no rotational deformity may be managed in a volar slab, again with careful follow-up during the first 10 days, those with uncorrected rotational deformity should be referred for open reduction and internal fixation.

Fractures involving the interphalangeal joints are liable to lead to residual stiffness and should be referred for consideration of reduction and fixation.

Phalangeal fractures should either be splinted by neighbour strapping or in a volar slab in the position of function.

Volar plate injuries

The volar plate is a fibrocartilagenous condensation of the joint capsule on the palmar aspect of the hand. Injuries to the volar plate occur as a result of a hyperextension force. In the majority of cases no bony injury is seen on the radiograph, on occasion a small fragment of bone is seen to be avulsed from the palmar aspect of the phalanx.

The initial management consists of neighbour strapping and gentle mobilization for 7–10 days. In a small proportion of cases the damage to the volar plate results in instability of the joint and in such cases operative repair is required.

Dislocations

Dislocations of the interphalangeal joints are common and in the majority of cases may be reduced by application of traction under a ring block. In a few instances it may be difficult or impossible to reduce the dislocation: this may be due to 'button-holing' of the head of the proximal bone through the capsule or volar plate; open reduction and repair may then be required.

Compound fractures of the terminal phalanx

Such fractures are common and result from a crushing injury. The nailbed is often lacerated in association with a comminuted fracture of the terminal phalanx. The nail should be removed under a ring block and the nailbed repaired. This will suffice to reduce the comminuted terminal phalanx. The nail may then be replaced. Some consider that prophylactic antibiotics should be used, others advocate treating only infected finger tips.

Lacerations

Bleeding from lacerations of the hand will usually resolve with the application of mild pressure and elevation. The temptation to explore a would to stop bleeding (except under controlled conditions with a tourniquet and adequate lighting) should be resisted in order to avoid damage to other structures.

A history of penetrating injury will suggest the possibility that tendons and nerves may have been affected. Such injuries are particularly common in the hand with glass cuts and in the fingers with knife cuts. It is sensible to radiograph any injury caused by broken glass to exclude a retained fragment. Experience has shown that failure to follow this simple rule, even when the wound seems trivial, leads to embarrassment on occasion.

Observation of the hand and position of the fingers will often reveal the presence of an underlying complete tendon injury. In the presence of isolated nerve or incomplete tendon injuries, the location of the wound is a guide to the structures likely to be involved.

Tendons

Lesions

1. Flexor digitorum superficialis (FDS). The tendons run superficially through the carpal tunnel and the palm to insert in the base of the middle phalanx of the four fingers. They act to flex the proximal interphalangeal joint (PIPJ), an action shared with flexor digitorum profundus (FDP). The integrity of FDS can be confirmed by demonstrating active flexion at the PIPJ for a particular digit by asking the patient to flex the finger while the examiner holds the other three digits in full extension. Immobilizing the other three digits overcomes the tendency of FDP to flex the PIPJ. This manoeuvre acts to inactivate the flexion at the PIPJ due to FDP, because FDP arises from a common muscle mass.

2. Flexor digitorum profundus. The tendons of FDP run deep to those of FDS to insert in the distal phalanx of each finger. FDP produces flexion at both PIPJ and distal interphalangeal joint (DIPJ). The intact FDP tendon will produce flexion at the DIPJ with the PIPJ held in extension; since no other tendon acts on this joint, any degree of active flexion at this joint demonstrates the integrity of the tendon.

3. Extensor tendon. Complete laceration of the extensor tendon is usually evident on observation of the relaxed hand. The affected finger is held in flexion by the unopposed action of the flexors when compared to the unaffected fingers. Active testing of extension is made difficult because the intrinsic muscles of the hand contribute to extension at the meta-carpo phalangeal joint (MCPJ). The hand should be held palm down against a firm flat surface and the patient asked to extend the digits. The ability to hyperextend at the MCPJ suggests that the extensor tendon is intact.

Incomplete laceration of any of the tendons may not be evident on examination. The tendon is liable to completely divide at some later stage. To overcome this problem, it is wise to explore all penetrating wounds of the hand over vulnerable areas to exclude partial division of tendons.

4.   Thumb. Division of the flexor pollicis longus tendon leads to loss of active flexion at the interphalangeal joint. Division of either or both extensors of the thumb leads to a reduction or loss of extension at the interphalangeal joint.

Management

Flexor tendons should be repaired under full aseptic technique in theatre by an experienced hand surgeon. Extensor tendon injuries on the dorsum of the hand may be repaired under clean conditions in the A&E Department. The repaired tendon is then protected by placing the hand in a volar slab for 3–4 weeks. In the case of extensor injuries to the thumb, a Bennet's plaster may be used.

1.   Acute rupture of the central slip of the extensor tendon. Closed injury to the extensor expansion over the dorsum of the PIPJ may lead to rupture of the central slip with corresponding lateral slipping of the lateral bands. In the acute phase, extension is lost at the PIPJ, later the characterisitc *boutonnière* deformity develops, with fixed flexion at the PIPJ and hyperextension at the DIPJ. The PIPJ should be splinted in extension, because of the tendency of this injury to progress, and the patient should be referred to a hand surgeon for follow-up.

2.   Mallet deformity. Forced flexion at the DIPJ may result in local rupture of the extensor tendon, this may or may not be associated with avulsion of a portion of the base of the distal phalanx. The finger tip is flexed and lacks active extension. This injury is treated by splintage of the DIPJ in full extension using a mallet splint for a period of 6 weeks. With early splintage the results are good. Delayed presentation leads to a poorer outcome with loss of active extension at the joint.

Nerves

Anatomy and examination   There is considerable variation in the cutaneous distribution of the median and ulnar nerves in the hand.

- The ulnar nerve supplies the little finger and the ulnar border of the ring finger in the hand.
- The median nerve supplies the radial border of the ring finger, the middle and index fingers and the thumb.
- The radial nerve supplies a small area of the dorsum of the first web space.

In the early phase of nerve injuries patients may experience difficulty in appreciating sensory loss, this is particularly so with ulnar nerve lesions.

The most reliable simple test of an intact cutaneous nerve supply is assessment of light touch and pinprick sensation. The 'Biro' test may also be used. A plastic pen is gently drawn across the ulnar and radial aspect of each digit, commencing on the side of the hand furthest from the suspected lesion. In the presence of an intact nerve supply resistance to movement will be encountered. If the nerve is divided, the sympathetic supply to the skin of the region supplied will be interrupted and sweating will cease. The pen will be felt to glide without resistance over the skin. In addition to loss of sensory innervation the motor supply of the nerve should be evaluated:

1.   Ulnar nerve. The ulnar nerve supplies the short abductor of the little finger and the first dorsal interosseous muscle. Loss of motor supply to these muslces can be tested by asking the patient to abduct the fingers against resistance. In the presence of an intact ulnar nerve the above-mentioned muscles can be felt to contract over the hypothenar border of the hand.

The adductor pollicis is the last muscle to be supplied by the ulnar nerve during its course through the hand. Loss of nerve supply to this muscle anywhere along its course results in the inability of the patient to keep the thumb tightly adducted against the index finger when the examiner applies an abducting force to the thumb.

2.   Median nerve. The abductor pollicis brevis is the only muscle in the hand invariably supplied by the median nerve. The thumb is placed in abduction and the patient is asked to maintain it there against an adducting force applied by the examiner. In the presence of a median nerve lesion the patient cannot maintain the thumb in abduction. If the thenar eminence is palpated at the same time, no contraction of abductor pollicis brevis can be felt.

3. Digital nerves. Digital nerve lesions should be suspected in any laceration to the finger, particularly in the presence of arterial bleeding. The 'Biro' test will confirm the presence of a nerve lesion.

Management   All nerve lesions or suspected nerve lesions should be referred for early exploration under tourniquet and with adequate light. The results of early repair are good, delayed repair gives poorer results, especially in the case of ulnar nerve lesions.

Amputations

Finger-tip injuries with loss of tissue distal to the nailbed may be treated conservatively, particularly in younger children. Contused, ragged lesions involving significant exposure of bone or more proximal finger tip injuries, particularly in adults, are best treated by primary debridement and coverage by one of the several available flap methods.

The possibility of re-implantation of clean amputated digits or parts of a digit proximal to the DIPJ should always be considered. In such cases early consultation with the local hand surgeon should be carried out. The amputated part should be wrapped in saline-soaked gauze, placed in a plastic bag and placed on ice (the amputated part should not be placed in direct contact with ice). The amputated part should accompany the patient to the referral centre.

Infections

The general principle of wound management is that superficial spreading infection should be treated by antibiotics initially, but that abscesses require drainage.

Staphylococcus aureus is the most common organism to be implicated in hand infections. The majority of staphylococcal infections encountered in clinical practice are sensitive to flucloxacillin and erythromycin. The presence of lymphangitis should suggest the possibility of streptococcal infection and penicillin V should be added.

Paronychia   Infection of the nailfold is common. In the majority of cases such infection resolves spontaneously with rest and analgesia, or progresses to local abscess formation. Once a local abscess has formed, simple drainage and appropriate antibiotic therapy are all that are generally required to resolve the infection.

Pulp infection

Occasionally a paronychia will progress to a pulp space infection. This is characterized by a red, swollen, exquisitely tender pulp. The patient will complain of throbbing pain, particularly at night. In the early stages treatment with oral antibiotics combined with elevation and analgesia may suffice to resolve the infection. In some cases drainage of the pulp space through a longitudinal incision may be required.

Tendon sheath infection

In a few cases a pulp space infection will progress proximally to involve the flexor tendon sheath. Infection of the flexor tendon sheath is characterized by pain on passive extension of the digit involved. While early cases may respond to elevation and antibiotics, all cases should be referred to a hand surgeon as established infection is likely to require open drainage of the tendon sheath: appropriate referral should therefore be made early if there is any suspicion of flexor sheath involvement. Complications include web-space infections and residual stiffness of the affected digit.

Web-space infections

These are characterized by swelling of the hand, dull throbbing pain (sufficient to keep the patient awake at night) and, in extreme cases, systemic upset. Clinically the affected hand is red and swollen. Even minor degrees of passive flexion will elicit severe pain. Treatment is by wide-open drainage of the affected deep tissue spaces, elevation and the use of systemic antibiotics.

Clench fist injuries

These are injuries to the knuckle, frequently extending to the MCPJ, caused by a punch to the mouth and involving a puncture wound by a human tooth to the MCPJ. Such injuries deserve their sinister reputation. The injury will frequently involve a fracture of the distal metacarpal and contamination of the MCPJ with a variety of organisms, including *Pasteurella*, actinomycites and *Bacteroides*. Treatment involves early exploration of the wound for a foreign body, and debridement, elevation and broad-spectrum systemic antibiotics. Radiography for a foreign body may be appropriate if there is considered to be a possibility of foreign body (usually a fragment of tooth). Stiffness of the MCPJ is a common sequela.

Non-bacterial infections of the hand occasionally cause confusion; these include herpetic infections of the terminal phalanx and orf, cutaneous anthrax is now rare.

Further reading

Wilson GR, Nee PA, Watson JS. *Emergency Management of Hand Injuries.* Oxford Handbooks of Emergency Medicine. Oxford: Oxford University Press, 1997.

Related topics of interest

Antibiotic therapy (p. 36)
High-pressure injection injuries (p. 136)
Human and animal bites (p. 147)
Nailbed injuries (p. 207)
Peripheral nerve injuries (p. 234)
Wrist injuries (p. 324)

HEAD INJURIES

Estimates of the incidence of head injury vary, but approximately 10% of patients attending an A&E Department do so with a head injury. Of one million head injuries each year, half that number happen to children. Two hundred patients per 100 000 population attend A&E each year with a head injury. Road-traffic accidents account for 25% of head injuries (36% in children) but approximately 60% of head injury deaths. Head injuries are twice as common in men as in women.

Categories

Head injuries may be divided as follows:

- Scalp.
- Skull.
- Brain.

The term 'head injury', by convention has come to mean brain injury and these injuries are divided into:

1. Primary (direct).

- Cortical contusions/lacerations.
- Diffuse white matter lesions.

Primary injuries may be closed or open and the tissue damage caused is not improved by treatment. Diffuse white matter lesions result from mechanical shearing forces with disruption and tearing of axons.

2. Secondary.

- Hypoxia.
- Hypovolaemia.
- Cerebral oedema.
- Infection.

Clinical management based on the vigorous management of airway, breathing and circulation must be directed to reducing the devastating effects of secondary injury.

Initial assessment

When taking a head injury history the following details must be obtained:

- Nature and timing of the accident.
- Use of alcohol or drugs.
- History of amnesia or loss of consciousness.
- Presence of headache or vomiting.
- Presence of fits.
- Other concurrent medical conditions.
- Availability of support at home.

Particular attention should be paid to the timing and duration of unconsciousness and of amnesia. The duration of post traumatic amnesia (PTA) correlates well with the severity of diffuse brain disease (retrograde amnesia is of less value).

The physical examination should determine:

- Conscious level, Glasgow Coma Score (GCS).
- Presence of signs of basal skull fracture.
- Bruises, lacerations to the scalp.
- Pupillary responses.
- Examination of the limbs.
- Cranial nerves (including visual acuity and fundi).
- BM stix®.

Indications for skull X-ray following initial patient assessment include:

- A history of unconsciousness or amnesia at any time.
- Impaired conscious level.
- Focal neurological deficit.
- Scalp bruising, haematoma or suspected penetrating injury.
- Alcohol intoxication.
- Difficulty in patient assessment (e.g. children, the handicapped).
- Cerebrospinal fluid (CSF) rhinorrhoea or otorrhoea.
- Severe (and worsening) headache.
- Vomiting, especially in children (who are 'allowed' to vomit once).

A high suspicion of head injury complicating another medical condition (e.g. epilepsy) should always be maintained. Never assume that an altered conscious level in someone who is intoxicated is due to alcohol.

Simple scalp laceration is not an indication for skull X-ray.

The risk of intracranial haematoma depending on the presence or absence of skull fracture in an altered level of consciousness is:

- Orientated with no skull fracture   1 in 6000.
- Disorientated with no skull fracture   1 in 120.
- Orientated with skull fracture   1 in 32.
- Disorientated with skull fracture   1 in 4.

Admission

Indications for admission are given below:

- Loss of consciousness.

- Altered conscious level at the time of assessment.
- Post-traumatic fit.
- Focal neurological signs or symptoms.
- Clinical or radiological evidence of skull fracture.
- Severe headache and/or vomiting.
- Extensive scalp laceration.
- Inadequate support or supervision at home.
- Difficulty in assessment.
- Haemophilia, warfarin etc.
- PTA > 5 min or no recall of the incident.

Despite this list, there will always be a number of patients who do not 'fit the criteria' for admission but do not 'feel right'. Where there is any doubt, these patients should be admitted.

CT scanning

Indications for CT scanning may be divided into those for immediate scanning and those for delayed scanning:

1. *Indications for an immediate CT scan.*

- Unconscious after resuscitation (GCS < 8). These patients have a 40% chance of intracranial haematoma.
- Decreased conscious level (GCS 8–13) with skull fracture.
- Deterioration in conscious level with progression to coma.

2. *Indications for a delayed CT scan.*

- Drowsiness or disorientation with skull fracture.
- Skull fracture with focal deficit.
- GCS 9–13 with focal deficit with or without skull fracture.

Other indications for CT scanning include patients requiring ventilation and patients requiring a general anaesthetic for orthopaedic (or other) surgery.

Definitive management

The vast majority of patients admitted to hospital following a head injury will require only observation. The management of more serious cases will depend on the presence or absence of neurosurgical facilities. Indications for transfer to neurological care include:

- Continuing neurological deterioration.
- Persisting unconsciousness (GCS ≤ 8) following resuscitation.

- Altered conscious level with skull fracture.
- Focal neurological deficit.
- Compound depressed skull fracture.
- Head injured patient requiring ventilation.

If it is necessary to transfer a deteriorating patient to neurosurgical facilities in another hospital, the patient should be anaesthetized, paralysed and ventilated *before* transfer. Similarly the patient should be stable following resuscitation before transfer is considered. The mortality of patients arriving at neurosurgical facilities with hypotension is approximately 75%, with hypoxia mortality is 60%. Tight cervical collars obstruct venous return, thereby raising intracranial pressure, and should be removed as soon as it is safe to do so.

Intracranial bleeding

1. Extradural. Extradural haematoma is most commonly temporal, 90% of adult patients with an extradural haematoma will have a demonstrable skull fracture (60–70% in children). The injury is often minor and there may have been no loss of consciousness. Classically a lucid interval is followed by a declining conscious level. Other features include contralateral weakness, ipsilateral pupillary signs and dysphasia. Treatment is surgical (preferable following a CT scan) with mannitol or frusemide being given as a holding measure if there is any delay.

2. Subdural. There are two main categories for this type of haematoma:

- Acute: usually secondary to severe primary brain injury.
- Subacute: occurs from ruptured bridging veins and is therefore more common in patients with pre-existing cerebral atrophy (alcoholics, the elderly). Diagnosis and localization are both difficult and CT scanning is required. Treatment is surgical.

3. Intracerebral. Intracerebral haemorrhages are usually due to coup or contra-coup injuries and may occur together with subdural haematoma. Deterioration is usually gradual over several days, the patient usually being ill to begin with. Diagnosis is by CT scan and management is conservative unless deterioration suggests the need for surgical evacuation of the haemorrhage.

Skull fractures

All compound depressed skull fractures should be surgically explored. Complications of skull fracture include:

- Intracranial haematoma.
- Cerebrospinal fluid fistula.
- Cranial nerve injury.
- Cosmetic deformity.
- Aerocoele.
- Post-concussion syndrome.
- Post-traumatic epilepsy.
- Meningitis.
- Hydrocephalus.

The possibility of non-accidental injury (NAI) should always be considered in children with skull fractures, and if the fracture is large, a 3 month review will be necessary to exclude a growing fracture with skull vault deficit. The threshold for admitting children should be lower than for adults.

Persisting symptoms following head injury

Physical symptoms persisting after head injury include:

- Headache.
- Pain or paraesthesia at the site of a scalp wound.
- Increased frequency of migraine attacks in previous migraine sufferers.
- Neck pain.
- Dizziness and vertigo.
- Vomiting.
- Oto/rhinorrhoea.
- Anosmia.

Psychological symptoms include:

- Tiredness.
- Instability.
- Sleep disturbance.
- Tension.
- Restlessness.
- Reduced concentration.
- Depression.
- Panic attacks.

Further reading

Currie DG. *The Management of Head Injuries*: Oxford Handbooks in Emergency Medicine. Oxford: Oxford University Press, 1993.

Related topics of interest

HEPATITIS B

The hepatitis B virus is a DNA virus, 42 nm in diameter. It is transmissible by all blood components and products except pasteurized albumin. The prevalence of hepatitis B surface antigenaemia in the UK is approximately 0.2% of the general population. Most antigen-positive patients give no history of having had clinical disease. The average incubation period is 40–180 days (commonly 60–90 days).

Mode of transmission

- Person to person. Percutaneous and permucosal exposure to infected body fluids (for a list of at-risk body fluids see the chapter on HIV infection), including transmission via tattoo or acupuncture needles.
- Parenterally. Unscreened blood, blood components or blood products (transmission via screened products occasionally occurs due to low levels of HBsAg).
- Vertical transmission: mother to baby.
- Sexual transmission: homosexual or heterosexual.

Clinical course of patients infected with hepatitis B virus

- 25% will develop an acute hepatitis of which 1% will die, the rest making a full recovery.
- 65% will have a transient subclinical infection before making a complete recovery.
- 10% will develop chronic hepatitis B infection (more common in children than adults).

Of those developing chronic hepatitis B infection:

- 10–30% will develop chronic hepatitis which may progress to cirrhosis or hepatocellular carcinoma.
- 70–90% will become healthy HBsAg carriers (some may eventually progress to cirrhosis or hepatocellular carcinoma).

Chronic carriers (those who are HBsAg positive or have hepatitis B virus DNA in their serum) may seroconvert when treated with α-interferon.

High-risk groups

- Intravenous drug abusers.
- Prostitutes.
- Sexual contacts of carriers.
- Health-care workers.
- Homosexual men.
- Those living in or originating from endemic areas. The prevalence in Africa, the Middle East and South-East Asia may be as high as 10–15%.

Clinical features of acute hepatitis B infection

1. *Prodromal phase (1–2 weeks)*
- Nausea and vomiting.

- Diarrhoea.
- Anorexia.
- Malaise.
- Headache.
- Low-grade fever.
- Upper abdominal discomfort.
- Urticarial or maculopapular rash.
- Polyarthritis.

2. *Icteric phase*

- Jaundice.
- Hepatospenomegaly (10%).
- Lymphadenopathy.
- Acute hepatic necrosis.

Treatment

In most cases this is symptomatic, patients with acute hepatic necrosis require appropriate management in a specialist unit. Chronic carriers may be offered treatment with α-interferon. Contact tracing in cases of sexually transmitted disease should be carried out and hepatitis B-negative contacts should be offered immunization and immunoglobulin.

Prevention of hepatitis B infection

In the health-care setting all patients should be assumed to be hepatitis B positive and precautions against transmission should be taken. Universal precautions are recommended. These include:

- Hand washing with soap and water before and after patient contact.
- Use of gloves when contact with bodily fluids is anticipated.
- Gowns and facial visors or goggles if splashes are likely.
- Adopting a sharps policy: care with unsheathed sharps, no resheathing of sharps, disposal of sharps in a puncture-proof, impervious container, prompt management and reporting of needle-stick injuries.
- Use of airway adjuncts in resuscitation to avoid the need for direct mouth to mouth contact in resuscitation.
- Prompt cleaning and disinfecting of areas in which spillage of body fluids has taken place.
- Ensure that all staff are immunized against hepatitis B and that their immune status is known and up to date.

Recommendations for vaccination	• All health-care personnel (including emergency services).
	• Morticians and embalmers.
	• Travellers to endemic areas.
	• Homosexual men, bisexuals and prostitutes.
	• Intravenous drug abusers.
	• Patients and staff of long-term institutions for the mentally ill.

Recommendations for vaccination and immunoglobulin

- Staff with needle-stick injuries (if hepatitis immune status is unknown, consult local policies).
- Newborn babies of HBsAg-positive mothers.
- Hepatitis B-negative partners of HBsAg-positive patients.

Hepatitis B vaccination

Active immunization is with a genetically engineered vaccine. Three injections are given at 0, 1 and 6 months. Response to the vaccine being checked at 3 months after the last injection. An anti-HBs level of 100 miu/ml indicates immunity. A booster is required after 3–5 years as antibody levels fall with time (alternatively booster doses may be given in response to a measured fall in antibody levels below the therapeutic levels).

Poor responders are defined as those achieving an antibody level between 10 and 100 miu/ml after a full course of immunization. These may require a booster dose, usually with a different vaccine.

Non-responders are defined as those with an antibody level less than 10 miu/ml after a full course of immunization. These will require a repeat course. This is usually done with a different vaccine. A few non-responders will be found to be hepatitis B carriers. Non-responders who fail to respond to a second course and test HBeAg negative are able to perform invasive procedures.

A UK advisory panel exists to advise on the occupational aspects staff who are hepatitis B or HIV positive.

Further reading

British Medical Association. *A Code of Practice for the Safe Use and Disposal of Sharps.* London: BMA, 1990
British Medical Association. *ABC of Blood Transfusion.* London: BMA, 1992.
Joint Working Party of the Hospital Infection Society and the Surgical Infection Study Group. Risks to surgeons and patients from HIV and hepatitis: guidelines and

management of exposure to blood or body fluids. *British Medical Journal*, 1992; **305:** 1337–43.

Kumar P, Clarke M. *Clinical Medicine*. London: Ballière Tindall, 1994.

Recommendations of the Advisory Group on Hepatitis. UK Health Departments. *Protecting Health Care Workers and Patients from Hepatitis B*. London: HMSO, 1993.

Related topics of interest

HEPATITIS C

The hepatitis C virus was discovered in 1988. It is a single-stranded RNA virus with six subtypes. Types I, II and III are seen in Europe, type IV occurs in the Far East. Hepatitis C is one of the viruses associated with non-A, non-B hepatitis. It accounted for 70–90% of post-transfusion hepatitis in hepatitis B-tested blood before the introduction of testing for hepatitis C in donated blood in 1991. Hepatitis C currently accounts for about 4% of post-transfusion hepatitis. The true incidence of hepatitis C in the UK population is unknown but is estimated to be 0.2–1%.

Transmission

Transmission is principally by the parenteral route, either from contaminated blood, blood products, or by contaminated needles (intravenous drug abusers, tattooing or acupuncture). Sexual transmission and vertical transmission (mother to child) appear to be uncommon.

Clinical features of acute hepatitis C infection

Unlike hepatitis A or B, the acute phase of hepatitis C infection may be very mild, a flu-like illness may occur with the following symptoms:

- Lethargy.
- Low-grade fever.
- Malaise.
- Backache.
- Nausea.
- Arthralgia.

Only about 10% of patients develop jaundice. The incubation period is 14–180 days, commonly 42–63 days. The mortality of the acute phase is about 1–2% and is due to fulminant hepatic necrosis.

Complications of hepatitis C infection

Approximately 80% of those acutely infected with hepatitis C will develop chronic infection, of which 10–20% will develop cirrhosis within 5–30 years; 10% of these will progress to hepatocellular carcinoma. Because of the high progression to chronic carrier status and the high complication rate in carriers, liver biopsy is recommended for those testing positive for hepatitis C. Up to 70% of patients will show evidence of chronic active hepatitis on liver biopsy. Grading of the histological changes can be used to guide treatment and follow-up.

Treatment

Approximately 25% of carriers show a sustained response to α-interferon treatment, although the long-term efficacy of this treatment in preventing progression to cirrhosis and hepatocellular carcinoma is unknown.

Prevention of hepatitis C   Screening of blood and blood products for hepatitis C has significantly reduced the incidence of post-transfusion hepatitis. Universal precautions should be adopted by all health-care staff when handling blood and body fluids of infected patients (see chapters on HIV and hepatitis B virus). There is currently no vaccine against hepatitis C.

Further reading

Booth R. Hepatitis C. *Professional Nurse*, 1997; **12** (4): 287–90.
Dusheiko GM, Khakoo S, Grellier L. A rational approach to the management of hepatitis C infection. *British Medical Journal,* 1996; **312:** 357–64.
Kumar P, Clarke M. *Clinical Medicine.* London: Ballière Tindall, 1994.

Related topics of interest

HIGH-PRESSURE INJECTION INJURIES

High-pressure injection ('grease gun') injuries result from the high-pressure inoculation of oil-based paints, lubricants, animal vaccines or other substances into the tissues, usually of the hand. The original case report in 1937 described an injury due to inoculation from a diesel engine injector system. Since this first description many substances have been associated with the condition: paint, paraffin oils, diesel oil, petrol, air, water, moulding plastic, cement, mud, wax solvent and animal vaccines.

Mechanism of injury

A pressure of more than 100 p.s.i. (689 kPa) is required to pierce the skin: at such pressures direct contact between the gun and skin is not required. The inoculated material is forced through the deep spaces and into the flexor sheaths. Forty-five per cent of injuries result in the foreign material extending proximal to the carpal tunnel. Factors influencing the distribution of the inoculated substance include:

- Injection pressure.
- Volume of fluid injected.
- Site of injection.
- Depth of penetration.
- Anatomy of the local tissue planes.

Tissue damage in the early stages is caused primarily by ischaemia due to arterial spasm, arterial and venous compression and/or thrombosis. Later injury is due to a combination of ischaemia, chemical inflammation and abscess formation.

Clinical presentation and diagnosis

In the early stages of the injury there are few symptoms. Patients will present with a puncture wound over the distal part of the digit (typically the non-dominant middle and index fingers) which may exude the injected substance: there may be minimal or no swelling and no pain. At this stage the injury may appear trivial, indeed the patient may not be aware that he has sustained an injection injury.

Within several hours ischaemia and chemical inflammation intervene, the digit becomes swollen, pale, turgid, numb and painful. At this stage the diagnosis and severity of the injury are evident.

Management

The mainstay of treatment for the majority of such injuries is early exploration, debridement and decompression of the tissue spaces. Post-operatively the limb should be placed in a volar slab in the position of function meta-carpo phalangeal joint (MCPJ) flexed to 90° and interphalageal joints (IPJs) extended to 180°) and the limb elevated.

Prognosis Even with early adequate drainage and debridement, a proportion of patients proceed to amputation. Complications post-operatively include stiffness, recurrent episodes of chemical inflammation and neuralgia. There is no evidence that the routine use of steroids improves outcome. The following are associated with a poor prognosis:

- Delayed definitive treatment.
- Increasing volume of inoculant.
- Type of inoculant (paint is worse than grease).
- Increasing injection pressure.
- Secondary infection.
- More distal site of injection.

It is important to remember that workers using high-pressure injection equipment who are aware of the significance of such injuries may present early, before any evidence of injury, other than the puncture wound, is present. Such patients should not be discharged. They should be discussed with the local hand surgeon so that plans for early exploration or admission for observation can be made.

Further reading

Burke F, Brady O. Veterinary and industrial high pressure injection injuries. *British Medical Journal,* 1996; **312:** 1436.
Couzens G, Burke FD. Veterinary high pressure injection injuries with inoculations for larger animals. *Journal of Hand Surgery,* 1995; **20B** (4): 497–9.
Gelberman RH, Posch JL, Jurist JM. High pressure injection injuries of the hand. *Journal of Bone and Joint Surgery,* 1975; **57A:** 935–7.
Rees CE. Penetration of tissue by fuel oil under high pressure from diesel engine. *Journal of the American Medical Association,* 1937; **109:** 866–7.

Related topics of interest

HIP FRACTURES AND DISLOCATIONS

Hip dislocation

Hip dislocation can be either anterior, posterior or central. By far the most common is traumatic posterior dislocation. Eighty-five per cent of traumatic dislocations are posterior, produced by transmitted longitudinal forces along the shaft of the femur, for example in dashboard injuries in car occupants.

Posterior dislocation

Posterior dislocations are usually associated with posterior acetabular margin fractures. The leg is held adducted, internally rotated and slightly flexed. The leg is shortened.

Following confirmation of the diagnosis by radiography, the dislocation is reduced as soon as possible under general anaesthesia. Post-reduction CT scan is recommended to exclude entrapped bony fragments.

These dislocations can be classified as follows (Epstein classification:

- Type I, dislocation with minor chip fracture.
- Type II, dislocation with single large posterior fragment.
- Type III, dislocation with comminution of the posterior acetabular lip.
- Type IV, dislocation with associated fracture of acetabular floor.
- Type V, dislocation with fracture of the head of the femur.

Operative treatment is indicated for:

- intra-articular fragments;
- fixation of Epstein type II injuries;
- Epstein types IV and V fractures if spontaneous reduction does not occur on hip relocation.

In all except type I injury, where traction is maintained for 3 weeks, patients are usually maintained in traction for 6 weeks. Subsequent mobilization is commenced as soon as possible.

The patient's initial condition may preclude surgery, in which case, the hip should be relocated and maintained on traction until surgery can be performed.

Total hip replacements occasionally dislocate posteriorly and may be associated with sciatic nerve injury.

Rarely, the prosthesis may 'buttonhole' through the soft tissue, warranting open reduction and soft-tissue repair.

Anterior dislocation

Anterior dislocations of the hip are rare and may be associated with forced extension of the hip with the patient weight bearing (for example, something striking the back.) Associated neurological and vascular injury may occur. The hip is held externally rotated and abducted, and like the posterior dislocation, slightly flexed.

Following reduction, the hip is maintained on traction for about 6 weeks. Complications include joint stiffness, avascular necrosis and secondary osteoarthritis.

Central fracture dislocation

Central dislocations occur due to a blow or fall on to the side. The head of the femur is driven into the acetabulum, producing a fracture dislocation. This type of injury may result from a lateral blow to a pedestrian from a motor vehicle. Associated intra-pelvic injuries may occur.

Initial management includes manipulation and traction. Consideration should be given to surgical reconstruction following appropriate plain radiographic and CT assessment.

Fractured neck of femur

Femoral neck fracture is most commonly seen in elderly females and is one of a group of injuries particularly associated with osteoporosis (the others are Colle's fracture, fractured neck of humerus and vertebral body wedge fractures). As well as post-menopausal osteoporosis, fractured neck of femur (NOF) may also occur in chronic debility states, including alcoholism, and in an elderly population already at risk of trauma due to increasing instability and cerebrovascular disease. Pathological fracture due to malignancy may also occur. Femoral neck fractures are rare in patients with osteoarthritis of the hip, in whom intertrochanteric fractures are more common.

Fractures may follow a definite fall or only trivial trauma. Occasionally a patient reports falling to the ground, having sustained a fracture during a simple twisting motion of the hips.

The blood supply to the femoral head is vulnerable, there being very little or no supply via the ligamentum teres. The blood supply comes from anastamotic vessels at the base of the neck in the capsular retinaculum. These may be disrupted in fracture displacement.

Fractured neck of femur is classified as follows (Garden classification):

- Grade I, incomplete fracture (abducted impacted fractures).
- Grade II, complete fracture without displacement.
- Grade III, complete fracture with partial displacement – posterior retinacular attachment is maintained.
- Grade IV, complete fracture with full displacement, posterior component is completely free.

Healing therefore will rely on vascular supply and bony apposition (i.e. adequate reduction of the fracture).

Classically, the hip lies in external rotation with some shortening. However in grade I and grade II fractures, the limb may look normal and only be painful on attempted movement. Patients may walk on an impacted grade I fracture, with an apparently normal plain radiograph. Is a fracture present or not? A painful hip and a history of a fall is suggestive of bony injury. In this situation it is important to exclude pubic rami fracture, an ultrasound scan will confirm the presence of a haemarthrosis, and a bone scan will be 'hot' if a fracture is present. It is usually wise to admit these patients for investigation and mobilization even if the investigations are normal.

Treatment

Treatment is operative. Patients should be taken to theatre as soon as they are medically fit. A short period of medical optimalization and anaesthetic assessment may be appropriate. Attempts to treat the elderly conservatively with long periods of traction are almost invariably associated with a high mortality due to pulmonary complications, bedsores and all the other sequelae of immobilization.

The best practice of fracture fixation in femoral neck fracture is a matter of debate. Some surgeons opt to fix grade I and grade II fractures while undertaking hemi-arthroplasty for grade III and grade IV fractures. Other surgeons contend that the risks of non-union and avascular necrosis are not that great, and therefore fix all grades of fracture on the premise that an arthroplasty can always be carried out at a later date if necessary. In support of this philosophy, some evidence exists to suggest a higher mortality with hemi-arthroplasty compared to percutaneous fixation.

The principles of treatment are:

- accurate reduction;
- secure fixation;
- early mobilization.

In patients under 60, failure to achieve adequate reduction in a planned percutaneous procedure is an indication for open reduction, although in these circumstances some surgeons would opt for total hip replacement rather than attempting fixation.

Complications – general

These relate to pre- and post-operative immobility, and include:

- DVT and PE;
- chest infection;

- urinary retention;
- pressure sores.

Complications – specific

1. *Avascular necrosis*. Various incidences have been suggested, perhaps as high as 10% of undisplaced fractures and 30% of displaced fractures. The patient develops hip pain, and radiography confirms collapse. The need for treatment, total hip replacement, is based on severity of symptoms and the patient's physical demands.

2. *Non-union*. Failure to achieve accurate reduction together with poor vascular supply may produce non-union. Treatment will depend on the patient's age, quality of life, symptoms and physical demand.

3. *Osteoarthrosis.* Secondary osteoarthrosis may follow avascular necrosis. Total hip replacement is the treatment of choice.

Intratrochanteric fractures

These are extracapsular fractures, and concerns regarding blood supply do not therefore apply. Like intracapsular fractures, intratrochanteric fractures occur most commonly in women in the eighth decade of life. Once again, these fractures may be due either to falls or to twisting movements. The intratrochanteric region is a common area for secondary metastatic deposits.

Clinically the leg is shortened and externally rotated and the patient is unable to lift the leg.

Treatment

Intratrochanteric fractures can be divided into stable and unstable groups according to the configuration of the fracture. In unstable fractures, the medial cortex and lesser trochanter are fractured, losing medial support. Notwithstanding this classification, almost all fracture patterns can be effectively managed by the use of a 'dynamic hip screw'. If the fracture has occurred due to the presence of metastatic disease (pathological fracture), it may be necessary to fill any bony defects with bone cement. There is no place for conservative management, even in the unfit or unwell, as prolonged bed rest for traction is likely to result in fatal complications. As with intracapsular fractures, 24 hours of pre-operative optimalization is useful in frailer or sicker patients.

Complications	All the complications previously listed can occur, in addition, residual deformity and non-union are common. Occasionally the metalwork may displace in patients with poor bone quality, requiring an alternative form of fixation.
Multidisciplinary approach	In all fractures of the hip, the importance of a multidisciplinary approach, involving surgeons, physicians, nurses, occupational and physiotherapists as well as social workers and the general practitioner, can not be over-emphasized.

Isolated trochanteric fracture

Isolated trochanteric fractures can occur:

- the lesser trochanter by the pull of the psoas muscle;
- the greater trochanter by the pull of the abductor muscle.

Following short-term rest and pain relief, these patients can be mobilized.

Femoral neck fracture in children

These fractures are rare in children and are usually associated with high-energy transfer in road-traffic accidents. As in adults, there is a high risk of avascular necrosis, which is particularly related to the degree of displacement. Children can also suffer acute traumatic displacement of the capital epiphysis, this should be regarded as a surgical emergency, and be reduced and secured as soon as possible.

Treatment	Undisplaced fractures may be treated conservatively. Displaced fractures require closed reduction and fixation with a hip screw.

Further reading

Parker MJ, Prior GA, Thorngreen K-J. *A Handbook of Hip Fracture Surgery*. Oxford: Butterworth Heinemann, 1997.

Related topics of interest

HIV INFECTION

The human immunodeficiency virus (HIV) is a retrovirus, containing an RNA-dependent DNA polymerase (reverse transcriptase), first isolated in 1983. Two types of the virus are known to cause disease in humans, HIV-1 is the principal disease-causing type in the developed world, HIV-2 occurs principally in West Africa.

Incidence

The incidence in the general population is 0.05%. HIV antibodies are found in approximately 1/80 000 blood donations.

Clinical features

There are four clinically distinct phases of HIV infection:

1.   Acute seroconversion illness. A proportion of those infected with the HIV will undergo an acute seroconversion illness. This usually occurs 3–8 weeks after initial infection and is characterized by an acute illness lasting for 2–3 weeks with some or all of the following symptoms:

- Fever.
- Maculopapular rash.
- Lymphadenopathy.
- Diarrhoea.
- Joint and muscle pain.
- Sore throat.

A peripheral neuropathy or meningoencephalitis may occasionally occur as part of this illness.

During the acute phase of the illness the patient develops antibodies to the virus. Such antibodies are usually present 6–12 weeks after initial infection, although antibody production may be delayed for 6 months or more.

The patient may remain asymptomatic for many years, symptomatic disease manifesting itself 2–15 years after initial infection (the average onset of AIDS is 10 years after initial infection).

2.   Persistent generalized lymphadenopathy. During the asymptomatic phase of the illness some patients will have persistently enlarged lymph nodes, but no other symptoms. HIV antibody test will be positive at this stage.

3.   AIDS-related complex (ARC). The patient develops a variety of constitutional signs and symptoms, without developing the opportunistic infections or cancers which define full-blown AIDS. These signs and symptoms described in ARC include:

- Diarrhoea.
- Weight loss.
- Skin rashes.
- Night sweats.
- Low-grade intermittent fever.
- Oral thrush.
- Fungal diseases (e.g. tinea infections).
- Viral infections (e.g. shingles).
- Chronic fatigue.
- Lymphadenopathy.

4. *AIDS*. The diagnosis of AIDS relies upon the identification of specific opportunistic infections and/or opportunistic malignancies in the presence of a positive HIV antibody test. The infections include:

- *Pneumocystis carinii* pneumonia.
- *Toxoplasma gondii* encephalitis.
- Chronic diarrhoea due to cryptosporidia and microsporidia.
- Pulmonary tuberculosis.

The malignancies include:

- Kaposi's sarcoma.
- Undifferentiated B-cell lymphomas.

Patients will usually be grossly underweight and may suffer neurological and neuropsychiatric syndromes.

Transmission

HIV can be transmitted by the following fluids: blood, semen, tears, vaginal and cervical secretions, breast milk, wound secretions, pleural, peritoneal and cerebrospinal fluids.

Faeces, nasal secretions, urine, saliva, tears, sweat, breast milk and vomitus, in the absence of visible blood, have not been associated with the spread of HIV *in the health-care setting*.

Normal social contact is not known to spread the disease.

Methods of spread

- Sexual contact: heterosexual, bisexual and homosexual spread occurs, although woman to woman spread is uncommon.

- From blood products: transfusion of infected blood or blood products, accidental inoculation from contaminated sharps, from accidental splashes on to mucous membranes or on to broken skin. In the 1980s haemophiliacs became infected through contaminated factor VIII preparations.
- From infected injecting or skin-piercing equipment; e.g. intravenous drug abusers.
- Vertical transmission: from mother to child during pregnancy, labour or from feeding with infected breast milk.
- Spread from infected health-care workers to patients is rare, even during invasive procedures.

Control of infection

The incidence of HIV in the community is approximately 1/2000, therefore an average Accident and Emergency Department seeing 50 000 patients per annum may expect about one HIV-positive patient to attend every 2 weeks. The mainstay of prevention of infection in the health-care setting is the taking of universal precautions when handling body fluids or sampling for blood.

Currently in the UK universal precautions are not commonly used outside high-risk areas. In this instance identification of high-risk groups will allow selective use of universal precautions. Such groups include:

- HIV-positive patients.
- Homosexual or bisexual men.
- Intravenous drug abusers.
- Haemophiliacs who have received unscreened blood or blood products (most will have been diagnosed if HIV positive).
- Others who have received unscreened blood or blood products.
- Sexual contacts of the above.
- Children of HIV-positive mothers.

Particular areas are known to have a high incidence of HIV infection, particularly sub-Saharan Africa. Care should be taken when handling the body fluids of any patient who has visited this area (or any other high-risk area), particularly if he or she has received a blood transfusion or had sexual contact in that area.

Infection control procedures

The following areas should be identified in any infection control policy:

- Handling and disposal of sharps.
- Adequate protection of open wounds and mucous membranes in staff.
- Adequate cleansing and sterilization of instruments (or disposal of disposable instruments).
- Testing of blood and blood products and restricting the use of such products.
- Testing of organ donors.
- Adopting a policy for the management of spills of blood or other bodily fluids.
- Adequate and safe disposal of clinical waste.

Risk of infection through needle-stick injury

The risk of contracting HIV through a needle-stick injury from a contaminated source is less than 0.5%. The risk of transmission from contact of infected blood with mucous membranes or skin is lower than that from needle-stick injuries.

Duty of health-care workers and employers

Any health-care worker who suspects that they may be at risk of HIV infection should report their suspicion to their occupational health department and undergo appropriate testing. During testing they should refrain from any exposure-prone invasive procedure.

Employers have a duty to counsel workers prior to testing, to keep their knowledge of the employee's HIV status confidential (unless it is in the public interest to reveal such information) and to find suitable alternative employment for those found to be HIV positive.

The finding that an employee is HIV positive does not preclude continuing clinical work, although such work must be carried out under medical supervision.

Further reading

Adler MW (ed.). *ABC of AIDS,* 4th Edn. London: BMJ Publishing Group, 1997.

Related topics of interest

Hepatitis B (p. 130)
Hepatitis C (p. 134)

HUMAN AND ANIMAL BITES

Bites account for approximately 1% of A&E visits and may be broadly classified into those of human origin and those of animal origin. Dog bites account for approximately 200 000 injuries/year in the UK. Because of the possibility of associated sepsis, which on occasion may be life-threatening, all bites should be treated with care.

Animal bites

In the UK dog bites account for over 80% of all animal bites, the majority of the rest being cat bites, following by a variety of other animal species. In adults, most dog bites are to the extremities, in children 80% are to the face and scalp.

Organisms present in bite infections

Infections from dog bites are commonly caused by *Streptococcus, Staphylococcus aureus, Staphylococcus epidermidis and Staphylococcus intermedius*. Infections due to *Pasteurella* are uncommon and usually produce intense inflammation of rapid onset. Infection developing after 24 hours is usually due to *Staphylococcus* and *Streptococcus* species. The majority of such organisms are sensitive to the standard antibiotics, including flucloxacillin, cephalexin, erythromycin, or co-trimoxazole. A similar profile of common organisms is found in cat bites, but *Pasteurella* infections are more common. Cat bites may also transmit cat scratch fever, toxoplasmosis and Q fever.

The Gram-negative rods *Capnocytophagia* spp. are commensal bacteria in the mouths of cats and dogs. They are sensitive to co-amoxiclav, erythromycin, chloramphenicol and tetracycline. These organisms are slow to grow in blood culture but may be associated with overwhelming septicaemia with renal failure and peripheral gangrene.

Management priorities

There are several issues to consider when determining the optimal treatment of such bites. These include the need for:

- radiography;
- formal wound exploration and debridement;
- wound closure;
- tetanus prophylaxis;
- rabies prophylaxis;
- antibiotic prophylaxis.

1.   Radiography. X-rays may be required to exclude an underlying bone injury (particularly in bites by powerful dogs), or to exclude retained radiopaque foreign bodies (usually tooth fragments). The history of a crushing-type injury in proximity to a bone, particularly in the hand, is a strong indication for a radiograph of the affected part.

The routine radiographing of an animal bite in the absence of a definite history of likely retained foreign body is not warranted. In such circumstances retained foreign bodies are uncommon. Extensive tissue damage or infection unresponsive to standard antibiotic treatment are indications for radiography. The possibility of a retained tooth fragment should be included on the request form so that appropriate views and penetration can be obtained.

2.   Formal wound exploration and debridement. The majority of animal bites can be treated by local tissue cleansing, with or without local anaesthetic infiltration (the infiltration being into clean skin adjacent to the wound rather than into the wound itself). The management of the wound itself follows standard principles.

Formal exploration and debridement should be reserved for extensive wounds with gross tissue destruction or contamination or where vital structures may be involved. This would usually be in cases where a bite affects the face or hands.

3.   Wound closure. Animal bites which require closure should normally receive delayed primary closure, especially if there is evidence of tissue destruction or likely heavy bacterial contamination. Wounds of the face (including scalp and ear) which has a good blood supply, and where the best cosmetic result is required, may be closed primarily after thorough wound toilet and debridement. It has been suggested that wounds which are closed primarily should receive antibiotic prophylaxis. Injuries which are more than 8 hours old should receive delayed primary closure.

4.   Tetanus prophylaxis. The standard guidelines for tetanus prophylaxis should be followed.

5.   Need for rabies prophylaxis. Rabies is not endemic in the UK and is rare in domesticated animals in most of western Europe, the USA and Canada. The incidence of indigenously acquired rabies in the USA from domesticated animals was approximately one case per year in the 1980s. In the situation were a patient presents with an animal bite sustained abroad from an unknown animal, and where the animal has not been observed for signs of rabies, rabies prophylaxis should only be commenced on the advice of the local infectious diseases specialist. Such instances are rare and should be discussed on a case by case basis.

6. Need for antibiotic prophylaxis. There is no doubt that for high-risk injuries (e.g. deep injuries to the hand, deep puncture wounds or extensively contused bites with devitalized tissue or bone injury) and in elderly, immunocompromised or diabetic patients, prophylaxis is warranted. If antibiotics are to be prescribed, the most appropriate is co-amoxiclav 500/125 three times daily. For penicillin-allergic patients, doxycycline 200 mg daily (erythromycin for children under 12 or breast-feeding mothers) is recommended. These antibiotics will cover *Pasteurella* spp., *Streptococcus* spp., anaerobes, *Staphylococcus aureus* and *Capnocytophagia* spp.

However, controversy exists over the need for antibiotic prophylaxis for simple animal bites. A recent meta-analysis (Cumming, 1994) looked at double-blind trials where antibiotic prophylaxis was randomized. The relative risk for infection in patients given antibiotics compared to controls was 0.58 (95% confidence interval 0.39–0.86). The infection rate in controls was 9%. Therefore only 3.8% of all patients would have benefited from antibiotic prophylaxis, or only 1 in 26 of patients treated. The majority of those developing infections had only simple soft-tissue infections amenable to simple treatment.

Antibiotics should not be used as an excuse for poor initial wound management, which remains the mainstay of treatment of all bites. The majority of wound infections will become clinically evident within 24 hours; patients should be advised as to the signs of infection and to seek medical advice if they develop an infection. If antibiotic prophylaxis is required, it should be commenced as soon as possible with a simple agent. Preferably, the first dose should be given at the time the patient is seen.

Indications for antibiotic prophylaxis

Patient indications	Wound indications
Elderly	More than 8 hours old
Splenectomy	Crush injuries
Immunocompromized	Puncture wounds
Immunosuppression	Bony injury
Diabetes	Hand/foot injury
	Following primary closure

Human bites

These are usually the result of a sporting injury or violence. The principles for management are the same as for animal bites. Superficial wounds may be managed as outlined above, antibiotic prophylaxis is not required *except for wounds of the hand*. Deep wounds and wounds to the hand and face should be covered with appropriate antibiotics (see below).

Several important differences exist between animal and human bites:

Type of injury

Deep wounds are more common in human bites, particularly those of the clenched fist variety affecting tendons and joints of the hand. Such injuries can be devastating if not managed by early surgical exploration and debridement.

Appropriate radiographs should be taken in all cases where a human bite of the metacarpal region is suspected. Radiography may demonstrate:

- foreign bodies (teeth)
- bony injury
- air in joints

Organisms present in human bites

Mixed aerobic and anaerobic infections are more common in human bites, an average of five organisms are cultured from such wounds, although over 40 organisms have been found in human saliva.

Other potential infections

Hepatitis B, syphilis and rabies are transmissible by human bite. There have been reports of transmission of HIV by human bite, although saliva itself is considered to be a low-risk biological fluid for HIV transmission.

Antibiotic prophylaxis

For wounds of the hand, augmentin is recommended by some, although good results are to be had from the initial use of flucloxacillin or erythromycin with or without the addition of metronidazole. All high-risk wounds should be followed up or the patients advised to seek medical advice if signs of infection develop. Infection will usually become obvious within 24 hours. Patients who present with tissue infection should be considered for admission for intravenous antibiotic therapy.

Wound closure   Bites to the metacarpal area should be treated by delayed primary closure following thorough irrigation with iodine. Bites to the face and scalp, if presentation is not delayed, may receive primary closure.

Further reading

Cumming P. Antibiotics to prevent infection in patients with dog bite wounds: a meta-analysis of randomised trials. *Annals of Emergency Medicine,* 1994; **23** (3): 535–40.
Mellor DJ, *et al.* Mans best friend: life threatening sepsis after minor dog bite. *British Medical Journal,* 1997; **314:** 129–30.
Moore F. 'I've just been bitten by a dog'. *British Medical Journal,* 1997; **314:** 88–9.
Skinner D, *et al.* (eds) *Cambridge Textbook of Accident and Emergency Medicine.* Cambridge: Cambridge University Press, 1997.

Related topics of interest

HYPOTENSIVE RESUSCITATION

Controlled hypotension in trauma is not new, indeed our physiological evolution has been designed to compensate for hypovolaemia. Cannon *et al.* (1918) recognized that 'shock hinders bleeding'. During the Second World War and the years that followed, intravenous cannulation and fluid replacement became increasingly practical, and with the advent of paramedics undertaking intravenous cannulation on scene, there has been an increase in prehospital times with no improvement in outcome. The ATLS programme has advocated normotensive resuscitation with no evidence on which to base such a policy. Attention has now focused on the possibility that overvigorous fluid resuscitation may itself adversely affect outcome from trauma.

It is already accepted that outcome in ruptured aortic aneurysm is improved if pre-theatre fluids are kept to a minimum. Similarly, controlled hypotension has been used for many years in open prostatic surgery to reduce blood loss.

Pathophysiology

It has been postulated that intravenous fluids:

- By restoring normal perfusion pressures, wash away established clots, relax sympathetic venoconstriction and promote bleeding.
- Produce haemoglobin dilution and reduce the concentration of circulating clotting factors.
- Produce hypothermia.

The evidence base

The first controlled trial to suggest a possible protective effect from hypotension was published by Bickell *et al.* (1994). They compared immediate versus delayed fluid resuscitation in patients with penetrating torso injuries. The 'delayed' group commenced intravenous infusion in the operating theatre.

The results can be summarized as follows:

- Delayed patients (289), 203 (70%) survived.
- Immediate patients (309), 193 (62%) survived ($P = 0.04$).

Other features included:

- decreased incidence of coagulopathy in the delayed group;
- decreased incidence of complications, including ARDS and renal failure, in the delayed group;
- decreased length of hospital stay in the delayed group.

Bickell *et al.* concluded that 'aggressive blood pressure elevation prior to control of internal haemorrhage may actually be detrimental'. It should be noted, however, that this study looked only at penetrating trauma.

Hambly and Dutton (1996) undertook a retrospective study to compare actual with expected survival of patients receiving fluid therapy via the Rapid Infusion System (RIS™) at the R. Adams Cowley Shock Trauma Centre in Baltimore. Inclusion criteria were:

- haemodynamically unstable patients following trauma;
- patients undergoing surgery with associated major blood loss and haemodynamic instability.

Exclusion criteria were:

- patients with a high spinal cord injury;
- patients with significant brainstem dysfunction;
- patients admitted in cardiac arrest;
- patients with a history of recent myocardial infarction.

The study included both penetrating and blunt trauma.

The overall survival rate in patients receiving fluid via the RIS was 52.9% ($n = 437$), which was significantly less than expected (61.8%, $P < 0.001$). The survival of victims of penetrating trauma ($n = 225$) was not significantly different from expected (actual 56.9%, expected 60.1%, $P < 0.056$). The survival of victims of blunt trauma ($n = 207$) was dramatically different from expected (actual 48.8%, expected 63%, $P < 0.001$).

Using matched controls, patients who did receive fluids through the RIS were found to have a 4.8 times greater chance of dying than those who did not.

The average volume of fluid received by the RIS group in this study was 9724 ml. There was evidence to suggest that the marked excess mortality occurred in those patients receiving the greatest volume of intravenous fluids (in excess of 6000 ml). The author concluded that the paper presented enough evidence to warrant further studies that might lead to a change in attitude to the role of rapid infusion in trauma victims.

Discussion

If it is accepted that hypotensive resuscitation has a role to play in the management of the victim of trauma, then the second question clearly concerns the level of systolic blood pressure which is appropriate. It has been suggested, based on experimental data, that very low blood pressures (in the region of 40 mmHg) may permit adequate tissue perfusion. To extrapolate this to the clinical setting would require the availability of skilled continuous invasive monitoring, and most clinicians would feel that this degree of hypotension would carry unacceptable additional risks. A compromise is necessary and it is generally agreed that a blood pressure of about 80 mmHg (i.e. a palpable radial pulse) is probably appropriate.

Conclusion

It would seem that the best clinical practice in the light of current evidence is likely to be:

- Short on-scene times.
- Airway and breathing secured at scene, together with control of significant external haemorrhage.
- Intravenous access secured in transit or in the A&E Department such that transfer to definitive care is not delayed.
- Fluid resuscitation only to a level which ensures perfusion of vital organs (BP (80 mmHg or the presence of a radial pulse).
- Avoidance of unnecessary delays in the A&E Department in patients with uncontrolled internal haemorrhage.

It is likely that such a policy will be increasingly supported by evidence from the prospective trials that are clearly required in this field.

Further reading

Bickell WH, *et al.* Immediate versus delayed fluid resuscitation for hypotensive patients with penetrating torso injuries. *New England Journal of Medicine,* 1994; **331:** 1105–9.

Cannon WB, *et al.* Preventive treatment of wound shock. *Journal of the American Medical Association,* 1918; **70:** 618–21. Reproduced with discussion in: Greaves I, Ryan J, and Porter K, (eds) *Trauma.* London: Arnold, 1997.

Dick WR. Controversies in resuscitation: to infuse or not to infuse (1). *Resuscitation,* 1996; **31:** 3–6.

Hambly PR, Dutton RP. Excess mortality associated with the use of a rapid infusion system at a level 1 trauma center. *Resuscitation,* 1996; **31:** 127–33.

Pepe PE. Controversies in resuscitation: to infuse or not to infuse (2). *Resuscitation,* 1996; **31:** 7–10.

Related topics of interest

IMAGING

Obtaining the maximum information regarding a patient's injuries is a vital component of optimum trauma care. First line investigations, which must never delay appropriate resuscitation, require a skilled radiographer with experience of trauma cases. The role of the radiologist must not be forgotten and in many centres is an underused resource. Ultrasound, computed tomography (CT) and selected angiography all have a contribution to make in identifying and quantifying injuries and hence leading to prompt and appropriate intervention.

The initial radiographic survey is part of the primary survey and consist of radiographs of:

Cervical spine

All seven vertebrae must be demonstrated.
Check for:

- Alignment of the anterior vertebral bodies, posterior vertebral bodies and spinolaminar line.
- Pre-vertebral soft tissue swelling.
- Rotation of the facet joints on each other.
- Disc space symmetry.
- Bone fragments.

A lateral film with AP, odontoid peg and obliques should be taken as required.

Signs of instability.

- Compression of vertebral body > 25%.
- Kyphotic angulation of > 11°.
- Widening of the spinous processes.
- Widening of the facet joints.

Classification of cervical injury

1. *Hyperflexion injuries.*

- Anterior subluxation.
- Bilateral locked facet joints.
- Flexion teardrop fracture.
- Spinous process fracture (clay shoveller's fracture).

2. *Hyperextension injuries.*

- Hyperextension strain.
- Fracture of the anterior arch C1.
- Fracture of the posterior arch C1.
- Hangman's fracture.
- Anterio-inferior vertebral chip fracture.
- Chip fracture.

- Extension teardrop fracture.
- Laminar fracture.

3. Axial compression.

- Burst fracture.
- Jefferson fracture (fracture of the pedicles of C2).

4. Flexion–rotation injury.

- Unilateral facet dislocation.

5. Extension–rotation injury.

- Pillar fracture.

Chest

Check:

- Rotation and inspiration.
- Mediastinal contour. If necessary an erect film may resolve concern.
- Pulmonary and pleural shadowing.
- Rib fractures and fractures elsewhere.
- Gas in the mediastinum, pleural cavity and soft tissues.

Localized injury may hide further damage, for example fractures of the first two ribs have a risk of vascular damage. Fractures of the lower ribs are associated with splenic and hepatic injuries. Sternal fractures are associated with thoracic spine fractures and haemopericardium.

Pelvis

A supine AP X-ray may be supplemented by inlet/outlet views and oblique acetabular (Judet) views.

The pelvis is a bony ring. If one fracture is seen the presence of further injuries should be considered:

- Double fractures of the pelvic ring are classified by force of injury.
- Isolated fractures are seen in the pubic rami, iliac wings and sacrum.

Fracture classification:

- Lateral compression or inward rotation of the hemipelvis.
- Antero-posterior compression which disrupts the iliac wings, sacro-iliac joints and symphysis pubis (open book pelvis). This injury is associated with bladder and urethral damage.

- Vertical compression: one hemipelvis is displaced upwards in relation to the other. This is commonly associated with major haemorrhage from vascular damage.

Secondary survey films   Skull, spine, extremity films as required.

Complex imaging modalities   *1. Computed tomography* (CT) requires transfer of patient to the scan room. It is imperative that unstable patients are continuously monitored and supervised.

- Head injuries: indications include:
  - (a) Depressed consciousness/loss of consciousness.
  - (b) Focal neurological symptoms or signs.
  - (c) Fits.
  - (d) CSF from nose/CSF or blood from ear.
  - (e) Deteriorating neurology.
  - (f) Persistent signs/symptoms.
  - (g) Open or depressed fracture.
  - (h) Penetrating injury.
  - (i) Inadequate history or examination.
- Abdominal and pelvic injuries: computed tomography must be performed before peritoneal lavage to allow accurate assessment of peritoneal and retroperitoneal damage.
- Chest injuries: scanning is valuable in both blunt and penetrating injuries for assessment of mediastinal, diaphragmatic and major vascular and cardiac injuries.
- Spinal injuries: plain films are unreliable for assessing the extent and severity of spinal injuries. CT with reformatting is essential to demonstrate bony and soft tissue detail.
- Intra-articular fractures: CT scanning may provide important information about intra-articular fractures.

2. Ultrasound. This can be done at the patient's bedside. It is quick and does not involve ionizing radiation.

- Ultrasound is used with abdominal injuries to assess visceral and soft tissue damage. It can be repeated if required. It is of limited value if retroperitoneal damage is suspected.
- Soft tissue damage is established by ultrasound (e.g. muscle haemorrhage, tendon rupture and foreign bodies).

3. *Angiography.* CT has reduced the use of angiography in chest injuries. However, selective angiography and embolization now has a major role in the control of bleeding vessels.

4. *Magnetic resonance imaging.* There is no apparent advantage over CT for acute brain trauma. MRI is now playing an increasing role in evaluating the patient with acute spinal cord injury. It requires no ionizing radiation and no invasive lumbar or cervical puncture for contrast instillation.

Further reading

Raby N, Berman L, deLacey G. *Accident and Emergency Radiology.* London: WB Saunders, 1995.

Related topics of interest

INJURY PATTERNS

Many injuries can be predicted given a good description of the accident that caused them. This information may not be available from the patient and it is important therefore to obtain as many details as possible from the ambulance staff and others present at the incident.

Kinetics of injury

Injury is caused by the exchange of energy either as the body stops falling or as a moving object impacts with the body. Thus the energy transferred to cause injury is related to the kinetic energy of the moving object. Kinetic energy (KE) is related to the mass (M) of the body and to its velocity (V) by the following formula:

$$KE = MV^2/2.$$

Thus for a doubling of the velocity, the amount of energy that has to be dissipated increases by a factor of four. Comparing a front-end impact at 25 m.p.h. and 100 m.p.h., although the speed has increased by a factor of 4 the kinetic energy is 16 times greater. Newton's second law states that energy can neither be created nor destroyed, it must therefore be dissipated, and this produces the patient's injuries.

Road-traffic accidents

The following general information should be established:

- The speed of the car, and of the oncoming vehicle if one was involved.
- Location of, and degree of damage to, the vehicle, and particularly the passenger spaces.
- Use of restraints (seat belts and airbags).

Certain injury patterns are associated with particular vehicular impacts, these are discussed below. However, these recognized patterns should never mislead the clinician into not looking for any other possible injury.

1.   Head-on impact. In assessing the likely injuries and their severity, the presence of impact damage to the steering wheel and 'bull's-eye' deformation of the windscreen predict serious injury to the chest and head and cervical spine, respectively.

In a head-on crash, the driver slides forward until stopped either by a seat belt (beware chest and clavicular injuries) or by his knees colliding with the dashboard (resulting in injuries to the patella, knee, shaft of femur or posterior dislocations of the hip joint). Following this sudden stop, the body is thrown up and forward allowing the head to strike either the roof or windscreen of the vehicle. The body will then impact with the steering wheel causing chest injuries (blunt trauma to the lungs and rib fractures).

At the same time there is an accompanying hyperflexion of the cervical spine, which then becomes a hyperextension injury as the body falls backwards following loss of momentum. Potentially critical cervical spine injuries are therefore likely.

A history of ejection from a vehicle greatly increases the chance of both serious injury and death. Passengers within a vehicle may also suffer from impacts with other unrestrained occupants as they are thrown across or out of the vehicle. The use of airbags has, to some extent, led to a decrease in serious injuries in head-on collisions; however, if they are activated in minor shunts, facial and ocular injuries may result.

2. *Side impact.* In side-impact collisions, injuries occur to the nearer side of the abdomen as well as the upper and lower limbs on the side of the impact. Fractures to the pelvis and compression injuries to the chest also occur. It should be remembered that a passenger on a bench seat in a minibus effectively suffers a side-on impact if the vehicle sustains a head-on collision.

3. *Rear impact.* These accidents result in hyperextension and flexion injuries to the cervical spine as well as the possibility of thoracolumbar spine injuries. In practice, significant cervical spine injuries are extremely rare in low-velocity urban rear-end shunts, which usually occur when a vehicle fails to stop in sufficient time at traffic lights.

4. *Motorcycle accidents.* As the motorcyclist falls, he may either stay with his vehicle or be thrown over the handlebars. If he stays with the bike and is dragged along the floor, he may suffer crush and soft-tissue injuries, including degloving. If thrown clear, as the cyclist leaves the bike, he may trail his legs, leading to fractures of the tibia or femur from impact with the handlebars. Further injuries may then be sustained as the victim strikes the floor, and can be predicted from the way in which he lands. If he is halted by the kerb striking his shoulder, he may

suffer bony damage in this area (fractures and dislocations) as well as soft-tissue injuries caused by hyperextension or depression of the shoulder or humerus. Vascular and brachial plexus injuries may occur. Various types of cervical spine injuries can occur, depending on the direction and magnitude of forces passing along the victim's neck.

5. *Pedestrians.* Adults hit by cars tend to be thrown up on to the bonnet if hit full on, and then slide off as the car brakes. As the car strikes the lower legs, fractures of the tibia or ligamentous injuries to the knees occur. The hips and trunk then strike the bonnet, finally the head strikes the windscreen or the front edge of the windscreen surround.

Injuries to children are different in a number of ways; small children are often hit at chest or abdomen level by the car bumper. They may be thrown completely clear of the vehicle or may be carried along by the car, sometimes being dragged under the car as it halts.

Falls from a height

If the patient lands on his feet, the following injury pattern may occur as the impact of landing is transmitted upwards from the feet: calcaneal fractures, tibial plateau fractures, acetabular and pelvic fractures and hyperflexion injuries of the thoraco-lumbar and cervical spines. If the spine remains straight, multiple lumbar fractures with collapse may occur.

Blast and gunshot injuries

Blast and gunshot injuries are fortunately still rare in United Kingdom practice. It is important to remember that the victims of blast may be injured by the direct effects of blast, by impact with the surrounding environment and by flying fragments. When assessing the victims of shootings it should be remembered that the path of a projectile within a body can not always be predicted from the entry point and that these weapons can produce devastating injuries at some distance from the muscle track.

Burns

It is important to remember that many of the victims of fires will have escaped in difficult circumstances and may have sustained injuries in so doing. These should not be missed in the initial patient assessment.

Further reading

Greaves I, Hodgetts T, Porter K. Taking a trauma history. In: *Emergency Care: A Textbook for Paramedics.* London: WB Saunders, 1997.

Related topics of interest

INTRAOSSEOUS INFUSION

The intraosseous space gained popularity as a site for vascular access in children in the 1930s. It was initially described as a method for blood transfusion. The method subsequently became unfashionable with the improvement in methods of intravenous access. A number of authorities have recently suggested that intraosseous infusion is an acceptable alternative to other methods of circulatory access both in the pre-hospital environment and within the hospital. Currently its use is mainly limited to paediatric emergencies when immediate attempts at percutaneous venous access have failed. Although adult intraosseous needles are now available, their use has not been widely evaluated. A wide variety of resuscitation fluids and drugs can be given by this route. Success rates have been reported to be approximately 80% and the complication rate is low at around 1%. Intraosseous infusion should only be used in the short term until an alternative vascular route can be accessed.

Indications in trauma

Failure to gain quick access by an alternative route or if access by another route is expected to take longer than 2 min.

- Cardiopulmonary arrest.
- Major trauma.
- Extensive burns.
- Major haemorrhage.

Contraindications

- Ipsilateral fractures.
- Ipsilateral vascular injury.
- Infection at the site of insertion.
- Osteogenesis imperfecta.
- Osteoporosis.
- Multiple ipsilateral attempts.

Uses

1. Fluid administration. Crystalloid, colloid and blood products can be administered. If rapid fluid resuscitation is required then bilateral infusions should be considered with fluids given by bolus or under pressure.

2. Drugs. Most drugs can be given by the intraosseous route at similar dosages and rates as the intravenous route. They should be followed by a bolus of saline to speed entrance to the systemic circulation. Hypertonic solutions such as bicarbonate should be diluted.

3. Laboratory investigations. All routine investigations needed for the injured or burned patient including crossmatch, haemoglobin, electrolytes and venous pH can be done on bone marrow aspirated from the needle.

Anatomy	Diffusion occurs from the red marrow into venous sinusoids in the medullary cavity. These sinusoids drain into venous channels that leave the bone via emissary veins before entering the circulation. This process is slower in children older than five as the red marrow is gradually replaced by less vascular yellow marrow.
Physiology	Circulation times for drug administration have been shown to be similar to other routes for vascular access especially if a saline flush is given immediately following the drug. Rates of infusion have also been shown to be acceptable.

Insertion sites

- Anteromedial aspect of the tibia 2–3 cm (two finger breadths) below tibial tuberosity.
- Anteromedial aspect of the femur 3 cm above the lateral femoral condyle.
- Medial aspect of distal tibia superior to medial malleolus.

Equipment

- Intraosseous needle between 14 and 18 gauge (spinal or bone marrow needles can be used as an alternative).
- Local anaesthetic if the child is conscious.
- Extension set.

Procedure

- Identify anatomical landmarks.
- Clean insertion site.
- Infiltrate local anaesthesia down to and into periosteum if the patient is conscious.
- The skin is punctured, the needle is then advanced with a screwing action at an angle of 60–90°, away from the epiphyseal plate.
- Entrance into the medullary cavity is signified by a decrease in resistance.
- The position is confirmed either by aspiration of bone marrow (often this does not occur) or a fluid flush with no resistance. A heparin flush should be administered to prevent clotting.
- The needle is secured with tape in an upright position and an extension set attached.
- Infusions are given by positive injection using a 50 ml or 20 ml syringe.

Complications

- Osteomyelitis.
- Compartment syndrome.

- Fractures.
- Extravasation of fluids or drugs.
- Cellulitis, abscess formation, skin necrosis and pain.
- Epiphyseal injury (theoretical, has never been reported).
- Fat and bone marrow microemboli.

Further reading

Fisher DH. Intraosseus infusion. *New England Journal of Medicine*, 1990; **332:** 1579–81.
Paediatric Life Support Working Party of the European Resuscitation Council. Guidelines for paediatric life support. *British Medical Journal,* 1994; **308:** 1349–55.
Spivey WH. Intraosseus infusions. *The Journal of Paediatrics*, 1987; **111:** 639–43.

Related topics of interest

INTRAVENOUS FLUIDS

Isotonic crystalloids

Isotonic crystalloids remain the first-choice fluid for the initial resuscitation of patients who are shocked. It is suggested that they are replaced with colloid and blood in grades III and IV shock. The volume of crystalloid infused should be appropriate to achieve adequate perfusion, but is based on multiplying the estimated losses by a factor of three.

The composition of standard isotonic crystalloids is given below:

Saline 0.9% (N/saline)	Sodium	150 mmol/l
	Chloride	150 mmol/l
	Energy (kcal/l)	0
Saline 0.45%	Sodium	75 mmol/l
Dextrose 2.5%	Chloride	75 mmol/l
	Energy (kcal/l)	100
Saline 0.18%	Sodium	30 mmol/l
Dextrose 4%	Chloride	30 mmol/l
	Energy (kcal/l)	160
Saline 0.18%	Sodium	30 mmol/l
Dextrose 4%	Chloride	50 mmol/l
10 mmol/500 ml KCl	Potassium	20 mmol/l
	Energy (kcal/l)	160
Dextrose 5%	Energy (kcal/l)	200
Hartmann's solution	Sodium	131 mmol/l
	Chloride	111 mmol/l
	Potassium	5 mmol/l
	Lactate	
	Energy (kcal/l)	0

Hypertonic saline infusions

Recent enthusiasm for hypertonic saline infusion (hypertonic resuscitation), which it was hoped would have advantages in terms of smaller infusion volumes, has waned as studies have demonstrated no advantages to their use. This is predominantly due to the transience of such fluids in the vascular compartment. They can not therefore be recommended for clinical use. Early studies suggest that the combination of a hypertonic fluid with a hyperosmolar fluid may be of value in the treatment of shock. It has been postulated that the hypertonic fluid draws fluid from the extravascular to the vascular compartment and the hyperosmolar fluid acts to keep it in the circulation.

Other crystalloid infusion fluids

For information, the composition of these fluids is:

Saline 0.45%	Sodium	75 mmol/l
Dextrose 5%	Chloride	75 mmol/l
	Energy (kcal/l)	200

Saline 0.18%	Sodium	30 mmol/l
Dextrose 10%	Chloride	30 mmol/l
	Energy (kcal/l)	400

Dextrose 10%	Energy (kcal/l)	400

Dextrose 20%	Energy (kcal/l)	800

Dextrose 50%	Energy (kcal/l)	2000

Colloids

Colloids are standard fluids for the resuscitation of shocked patients. Gelofusine® and Haemaccel® are the most commonly used, albumin is expensive and has no advantages which might justify its use in place of cheaper fluids. Contrary to a popular myth, neither Haemaccel® nor Gelofusine® interfere with cross-matching unless given in enormous volumes.

Albumin 4.5%	Sodium	150 mmol/l
	Potassium	1 mmol/l

Gelofusine®	Sodium	154 mmol/l
	Potassium	< 1 mmol/l
	Calcium	< 1 mmol/l

Haemaccel®	Sodium	145 mmol/l
	Potassium	5 mmol/l
	Calcium	12.5 mol/l

Starches are enjoying renewed interest, as there is some research evidence to suggest that the large molecular weight molecules they contain might have a protective effect against the development of capillary leak syndrome. It has been suggested that this might be due to direct plugging of leaking capillaries by the large molecules as well as to a reduction in neutrophil binding to vascular endothelium.

Fluid requirements in children

As well as replacing any fluid lost during trauma, the daily maintenance fluids of children must be carefully calculated. The following regime may be useful. The normal daily (hourly) fluid requirements, to replace insensible losses, essential urine output and to maintain a modest diuresis are:

First 10 kg	100 ml/kg (4 ml/kg)
Second 10 kg	50 ml/kg (2 ml/kg)
Each subsequent kg	20 ml/kg (1 ml/kg)

Further reading

Advanced Life Support Group. *Advanced Paediatric Life Support.* London: British Medical Journal Publishing, 1993.

Related topics of interest

Advanced Trauma Life Support (ATLS) (p. 11)
Hypotensive resuscitation (p. 152)
Intraosseous infusion (p. 164)
Pneumatic anti-shock garment (PASG/MAST suit) (p. 238)
Vascular trauma (p. 317)

INVASIVE MONITORING

The introduction of non-invasive modalities of monitoring such as pulse oximetry and continuous end-tidal CO_2 measurement has reduced the need for early invasive monitoring in the acutely traumatized patient. The initiation of invasive monitoring should not interfere with the initial phase of resuscitation based upon clinical assessment and non-invasively derived parameters.

Direct arterial pressure monitoring

This allows for continuous, direct measurement of systolic, diastolic and pulse pressure. A catheter placed in the radial artery is connected to a pressure transducer which is in turn connected to a monitor. It is of particular value in low-output states when the standard indirect manual or automated sphygmomanometric method fails to measure blood pressure.

Complications.

- Arterial wall damage (e.g. intimal tears) and thrombosis.
- Embolism.
- Disconnection and haemorrhage.
- Sepsis.
- Tissue necrosis.

Central venous pressure monitoring

A catheter introduced through a central vein or via a peripheral vein placed such that its tip lies at the lower end of the superior vena cava or within the entrance to the right atrium is used to measure central venous pressure (CVP), either continuously using a monitor and electronic transducer or intermittently using a manometer. The transducer must be zeroed with respect to the surface markings of the right atrium. The most reliable route for central venous cannulation is the jugular route. Correct placement must be confirmed by obtaining a chest X-ray. CVP provides information on the volume status of the circulation which is of particular value when large volumes of fluid are to be administered in response to shock. Trends in CVP readings provide more information than individual readings. CVP gives indirect information as to the state of the myocardium and the need for inotropic support.

Complications. Jugular route:

- Air embolism.

- Carotid artery puncture.
- Brachial plexus injury.
- Phrenic nerve injury.
- Ectopic placement.
- Pneumothorax.

Subclavian route (complications more frequent than by the jugular route and correct placement less likely):

- Pneumothorax.
- Subclavian artery puncture.
- Air embolism.
- Thoracic duct puncture (left side).

The technique requires skill. The risk of pneumothorax, particularly when using the subclavian route, makes this technique unsuitable in the early phase of resuscitation.

Pulmonary artery pressure monitoring (Swan–Ganz catheter)

In general, CVP monitoring provides reasonably accurate information on the state of the myocardium by estimating right and left atrial pressures. The assumption that left atrial pressure correlates with right atrial pressure cannot be made in the following circumstances:

- Left ventricular failure.
- Pulmonary oedema.
- Chronic lung disease.
- Valvular heart disease.

In such circumstances the CVP may not be sufficient to titrate ionotropes against cardiac function, and in these cases a wedged pulmonary artery catheter (via an inflatable balloon) can be used to gain a more accurate estimate of left atrial pressure.

The catheter has up to four lumens, with the following functions:

- A proximal lumen which opens into the right atrium to measure CVP.
- A distal lumen which lies in a branch of the pulmonary artery and measures pulmonary artery pressure.
- A balloon lumen which is connected to a balloon just proximal to the tip of the lumen which can be inflated to occlude the pulmonary artery in which the distal lumen lies. When the balloon is inflated the distal lumen pressure reflects the left atrial pressure.
- A thermistor lumen which is connected to a small thermistor just proximal to the tip of the distal lumen

which is used to measure cardiac output by the thermodilution method.

The catheter is inserted via a central vein using a dilator. Placement may be difficult and time consuming. In practice most trauma victims are young with normal cardiorespiratory function and the CVP will provide sufficient information to allow accurate fluid replacement and ionotropic support in uncomplicated cases. The technique probably has no place in the early management of major trauma.

Complications. In addition to the complications of central venous cannulation, the following may arise:

- Arrhythmias on insertion.
- Knotting of the cannula in the right ventricle.
- Rupture and embolization of fragments of the balloon.
- Pulmonary infarction.
- Infection.
- Valvular damage.

There is much debate currently as to the value of pulmonary artery catheters in the management of the critically ill patient. There is little evidence that their use influences outcome, despite their obvious attraction in quantifying the management of fluids and ionotropes.

Intraventricular pressure monitoring

A bolt inserted into the skull is used to provide continuous measurement of intracranial pressure. This technique is usually confined to neurosurgical ITUs and is used in the management of raised intracranial pressure.

In addition to the above commonly used techniques is the technique of direct intravascular oximetry which has not yet been fully evaluated in the trauma patient.

Further reading

Aitkenhead AR, Smith G (eds). *Textbook of Anaesthesia*, 2nd Edn. Edinburgh: Churchill Livingstone, 1990.

Related topics of interest

KETAMINE

Ketamine, which is related to phencyclidine ('Angel Dust') was first described 32 years ago. It provides anaesthesia and amnesia, with analgesia at subanaesthetic doses, but its use can be complicated by the development of certain psychiatric problems known as emergence phenomena. The pharmacological properties of ketamine make it particularly suitable for pre-hospital use and anaesthesia for repeated short procedures.

Presentation

Ketamine hydrochloride, which is water soluble, is available in three strengths – 10 mg/ml, 50 mg/ml and 100 mg/ml. It can be given by intravenous or intramuscular injection.

Pharmacology

Ketamine produces the following pharmacological effects:

1. Central nervous system. Agitation, disorientation, restlessness and nightmares may occur on recovery ('emergence phenomena'). The incidence of these symptoms can be reduced by the avoidance of extraneous stimulation (noise and touch) during anaesthesia, together with the simultaneous administration of a benzodiazepine. The earlier the patient is disturbed during recovery, the higher the incidence of emergence phenomenon.

2. Cardiovascular system. The following changes will occur:

- ↑ blood pressure.
- ↑ pulse rate.
- ↑ cardiac output.

The rise in blood pressure, which may be quite dramatic, must not be mistaken for a response to fluid resuscitation as a subsequent fall in blood pressure may be seen.

3. Respiratory system. Pharyngeal and laryngeal reflexes are preserved, in comparison with other agents this has a protective effect on the airway. However, a patent airway can not be assumed and appropriate care must be still be taken. Ketamine produces bronchial dilatation and is therefore suitable for use in asthmatics.

4. Gastrointestinal system. Salivation is increased.

5. *Musculoskeletal system.* Muscular hypertonicity occurs, which may contribute to airway compromise.

Pharmacokinetics

Ketamine is mainly metabolized in the liver and the metabolites excreted in the urine.

Indications

- Analgesia or anaesthesia for short repeated painful procedures, such as dressing changes. Frequent use of ketamine may affect the patient's sleeping and eating patterns.
- Trauma anaesthesia. Because ketamine produces a rise in blood pressure, it may be particularly valuable in the shocked patient.
- Anaesthesia in difficult locations. Obtaining surgical anaesthesia by use of intramuscular ketamine may be particularly attractive if intravenous access can not be achieved.
- Because of its relative ease of use, ketamine is popular as an anaesthetic agent in developing countries.

Administration

The ideal route of administration is intravenous, particularly in the shocked patient where muscle perfusion may be inadequate at the time of administration, but may suddenly recover following treatment, producing delayed and inappropriate effects. Ketamine is safe at doses many times the therapeutic dose.

1. *Anaesthesia.* Dose: intravenous boluses, 2 mg/kg with additional doses of 1–1.5 mg/kg every 5–10 minutes; intramuscular, 8–10 mg/kg.

Care should be taken with all recommended doses of ketamine as the doses given for both analgesia and anaesthesia vary dramatically between authorities.

Following intravenous administration, ketamine produces anaesthesia in 30–60 seconds. A single intravenous dose produces unconsciousness for 10–15 minutes. Onset of anaesthesia following intramuscular injection takes 4–5 minutes, peak concentrations occur after about 20 minutes.

Administration of ketamine in an anaesthetic dose produces a state of *dissociative anaesthesia* characterized by:

- Profound analgesia.
- Amnesia.
- Cataplexy.

The patient's eyes may remain open. Due to the persistent increase in muscle tone and the cataplexy, the patient's limbs may remain in abnormal positions if so placed by the doctor administering the drug. Patients may mutter or make abnormal sounds.

2. *Analgesia.* Dose: intravenous 1 mg/kg. In lower doses than those used for anaesthesia, ketamine produces analgesia without loss of consciousness.

Side-effects

1. *Central nervous system.* As well as the emergence phenomenon described above, facial grimacing and athetoid movements may occur. Ketamine may affect the mental state in between 5 and 30% of patients. Raised intracranial pressure may occur and ketamine should therefore be used with caution in head-injured patients, although it has recently been suggested that this effect does not occur at analgesic doses.

2. *Cardiovascular system.* The hypertension and tachycardia it produces may be a relative contraindication to the use of ketamine in patients with hypertension or ischaemic heart disease.

3. *Respiratory system.* Transient apnoea may occur after rapid intravenous administration. Equipment for temporary respiratory support should therefore be available before induction of anaesthesia.

4. *Gastrointestinal system.* Excessive salivation may compromise the airway. In hospital practice, the use of an anticholinergic agent should be considered.

Safety

Currently ketamine is not a controlled drug, it is however a drug of abuse ('special K') and appropriate precautions should be taken to ensure its safety, especially during pre-hospital use.

Further reading

Aitkenhead AR, Smith G (eds). *Textbook of Anaesthesia,* 2nd Edn. Edinburgh: Churchill Livingstone, 1990.

Related topics of interest

KNEE: SOFT-TISSUE INJURIES

The knee is a complex hinge joint. In addition, a small amount of antero-posterior translation, as well as rotation in the form of terminal locking occurs. Stability of the knee is maintained by the intrinsic bony structure with interspersed menisci, and the cruciate and collateral ligaments in conjunction with musculo-tendonous stabilizers including the hamstring and quadriceps mechanisms. Common patterns of injury include internal mechanical derangements due to injuries, such as meniscal tears or loose bodies, and symptoms due to instability as a consequence of ligamentous injuries.

Presenting symptoms

The most common presenting symptom is pain, which is often localized. The classical symptoms of internal mechanical derangement are:

- Swelling.
- Locking.
- Giving way.

Swelling when due to an effusion, is usually delayed in onset, whereas that due to haemarthrosis is invariably immediate. True locking implies a mechanical block within the joint itself which may be 'unlocked' by appropriate manipulation. The classical position of locking is in approximately 30–40° of flexion. Giving way is due to inhibition of quadriceps mechanism.

Meniscal injuries

This is a common problem, often occurring in young sportsmen with a history of a rotational injury on a semiflexed knee. The patient typically complains that the knee is swollen, locks and gives way. Physical signs include joint effusion, tenderness in relation to the joint line over the meniscus, a positive *McMurray's test* (a palpable click on rotation at varying degrees of flexion), and a positive *Apley's compression test* (axial loading in the prone patient with the knee flexed to 90°).

The locked knee requires surgical intervention with arthroscopy. There is no merit in manipulation of the knee under sedation in the Accident and Emergency Department. This merely delays intervention by generating a wait for out-patient follow-up, and may exacerbate quadriceps wasting due to immobility and pain. Definitive meniscal surgery is required. It should be noted that acute meniscal tear can present as a haemarthrosis when there is a major disruption at the menisco-synovial junction. If this is the case, then surgical repair produces good results.

Whereas the results of open and partial arthroscopic meniscectomy are the same, the reduction of pain, early mobilization and non-invasive nature of the latter technique make it the usual treatment of choice. In general, patients with bucket-handle tears fare better than those with degenerative or flap tears of the menisci. There is an increased incidence of osteoarthritis in those patients who have undergone total meniscectomy.

Ligament injuries

Instability may be divided into instability on rotation (rotational instability) and instability on antero-posterior or medio-lateral movement (straight instability or abnormal translation). Combinations of these instabilities may be found. Ligament injuries of the knee are graded 1–3, where grade 1 represents a simple sprain without laxity, grade 2 partial disruption without frank instability, and grade 3 represents obvious complete disruption. It should be noted that a feature of partial injury is intense pain, whereas complete ruptures are often pain free.

Straight instability is seen in medial collateral (MCL), lateral collateral, anterior cruciate or posterior cruciate injuries. Rotational instability is a feature of antero-medial or antero-lateral injuries. Specific diagnostic tests are as follows.

Straight instability

	Test	Pathology
1. Medial	Abduction laxity tested at 30° of flexion	MCL injury
2. Lateral	Adduction laxity tested at 30° of flexion	Lateral complex tear
3. Anterior	Positive anterior drawer sign	Anterior tear cruciate
4. Posterior	Positive posterior drawer sign	Posterior cruciate tear

Rotational instability

	Test	Pathology
1. Antero-lateral	Positive pivot shift test	Anterior cruciate tear; injury to lateral capsular ligament
2. Antero-medial instability	Positive abduction stress test and positive anterior drawer test in external rotation	Anterior cruciate tear; injury to postero-medial capsular structures

The most common rotator instability is the antero-lateral instability with a *positive pivot shift test*, a palpable and visible shift of the tibia is seen between 20° and 30° of flexion as the knee is flexed or extended with the tibia held in internal rotation.

3. Complex instability. These result from a combination of rotator instabilities or straight and rotator instabilities.

Medial collateral ligament injuries

The medial collateral ligament comprises superficial and deep components and blends posteriorly with the posterior oblique ligament. Consequently, medial instability is often associated with postero-medial laxity also. The medial aspect of the knee is reinforced by components of the pes anserinus. The medial collateral ligament is the main restraint when the knee is flexed at 30°. When in full extension, resistance to valgus strain is provided by the anterior cruciate ligament. Injuries of the medial collateral ligament can be either partial or complete; complete injuries usually being painless. Partial tears are generally associated with intense pain.

A common pattern of injury includes the medial collateral ligament, the medial meniscus and the anterior cruciate ligament as increasing force is applied to the knee. This pattern of injury is known as O'Donoghue's triad. In view of the high incidence of associated injuries, patients with clinically complete or probably complete medial collateral ligament injuries should be referred for an orthopaedic opinion.

Lateral collateral ligament injuries

The lateral structures of the capsule of the knee comprise the fibular collateral ligament, the ilio-tibial tract and the patellar retinaculum, and are tested by varus stressing at 30° of flexion. The anterior cruciate ligament is the main restraining force in extension, and therefore when the joint opens in extension there is usually an associated anterior cruciate injury. The patient should be referred for an orthopaedic opinion.

Anterior cruciate ligament injuries

The anterior cruciate ligament is composed of antero-medial and postero-lateral bundles. The antero-medial bundle is slightly lax in extension and tightens in flexion whereas the postero-lateral bundle is tight in extension and slightly lax in full flexion. Thus each bundle may be injured separately. The anterior cruciate ligament provides the primary restraint to anterior subluxation of the tibia on the femur: secondary restraint is provided by the collateral ligaments and the posterior capsule.

Injury to the anterior cruciate ligament is often associated with sporting injury to an extended knee and a popping sensation may be described: traumatic haemarthrosis usually occurs. It should be noted that isolated injuries are rare and the injury is usually associated with antero-medial or antero-lateral rotatory instability and with meniscal pathology (see O'Donoghue's triad, above).

Should an isolated anterior cruciate ligament injury be complicated by loss of secondary restraint, a straight instability will be converted into a rotatory instability.

The most reliable test for anterior cruciate disruption is the *Lachman test* which is positive in 85% of cases. A positive test is indicated by anterior translation of the tibia on the femur at 25° of flexion. The result can be graded from 0 to 3+ where 0 is normal, 1+ is 0.5 cm of abnormal translation, 2+ is 0.5–1.0 cm of abnormal translation and 3+ is translation of 1.0–1.5 cm. In addition, the patient may have a positive *anterior drawer test* which is abnormal translation of the tibia under the femur with the knee at 900 and the foot fixed. It has been suggested that the Lachman test stresses the postero-lateral component, whereas the anterior drawer test stresses the antero-medial band of the anterior cruciate ligament. The pivot shift test will be positive when there is antero-lateral rotatory instability, but it may not always be detectable in the acute stage unless the patient is anaesthetized. Patients with anterior cruciate injuries should be referred for an orthopaedic opinion. Although the initial management is likely to be physiotherapy and rehabilitation, those patients with features of chronic instability, and especially those with a positive pivot shift test, may require reconstructive surgery, taking into account their age and predicted future physical requirements. The presence of a bony avulsion at the point of attachment of the anterior cruciate ligament is an indication for urgent arthroscopy and fixation, and is associated with a good prognosis.

Posterior cruciate ligament injuries

Injury to the posterior cruciate ligament is usually associated with a significant force being applied to the knee: the knee is often flexed to a right angle, as, for example, when the knee of a car-driver strikes the dashboard. Haemarthrosis occurs together with a positive *posterior drawer sign*. Occasionally there are associated bony avulsions, which if present improve the prognosis following surgery. Most patients cope well with posterior cruciate deficiency.

Further reading

Apley AG, Solomon L. *Apley's System of Orthopaedics and Fractures*, 7th Edn. Oxford: Butterworth Heinemann, 1993.

Related topics of interest

LAPAROSCOPY AND THORACOSCOPY IN TRAUMA

Laparoscopy in abdominal trauma

The technique of laparoscopy was first introduced in 1911, and has been in widespread use for cholecystectomy since the late 1980s. Operations now performed laparoscopically include adrenalectomy, hernia repair and gynaecological surgery. In the past few years, there has been increasing interest in the role of laparoscopy in the diagnosis and treatment of abdominal trauma. In some specialist trauma centres in the USA, laparoscopy is now accepted as part of the conventional diagnostic armamentarium in abdominal trauma. Like all laparoscopic surgery, laparoscopy in trauma must be carried out by experienced operators. It has been suggested that the use of laparoscopy might lead to a reduction in the incidence of negative laparotomies.

Other diagnostic options in possible abdominal trauma include peritoneal lavage, ultrasound scanning (USS), computed tomography (CT) and conventional laparotomy. Like ultrasound scanning, laparoscopy is very operator-dependent; unlike peritoneal lavage, it allows anatomical location of injury. Laparoscopy allows inspection of the retroperitoneum, and may allow the possibility of therapeutic intervention. Unlike CT scanning, it can be carried out in theatre, and thus may avoid potential delays in resuscitation.

Indications

The following indications have been suggested:

- Exclusion of occult intra-abdominal trauma.
- Exclusion or demonstration of abdominal penetration in gunshot wounds or stab wounds below the nipple line.
- Assessment of diaphragmatic integrity.
- Aid blood salvage for auto-transfusion.

Disadvantages

- High negativity rates: a negativity rate of 60% has been reported even in patients with gunshot wounds of the abdomen.
- Expense.
- Difficulty in assessing small bowel injuries.

Complications

- Penetration of intra-abdominal organs, usually bowel.
- Pneumothorax or tension pneumothorax via pre-existing diaphragmatic perforation.
- Gas embolism.

New techniques

Gasless laparoscopy has the advantage of avoiding the risk of gas embolism or pneumothorax as vision is aided by holding up the abdominal wall with slings and retractors rather than distending the peritoneum with gas.

It has been suggested that the difficulty of assessing lengths of small bowel can be overcome by performing a mini-laparotomy (4 cm) and examining the bowel by bringing it out through the wound a loop at a time. A further possibility is distension of the bowel with intraluminal CO_2.

Thoracoscopy in chest trauma

Like laparoscopy, the technique of thoracoscopy is not new. However, recent developments in video technology have made it a much more useful diagnostic and therapeutic intervention in thoracic trauma. It is likely that the more widespread use of thoracoscopy would reduce the frequency of exploratory thoracotomy; it is clear, however, that thoracoscopy is not a substitute for thoracotomy in major chest injuries with catastrophic bleeding.

Thoracoscopy with mini-thoracotomy may well represent an advance in the surgery of chest trauma, as arthroscopic-assisted surgery has aided the treatment of the injured knee.

Indications
- Investigation of blunt chest trauma.
- Assessment and control of persistent non-life-threatening intrathoracic haemorrhage.
- Assessment of diaphragmatic integrity.
- Removal of organizing haematoma (delayed).
- Removal of foreign bodies.

Disadvantages
- Deflation of the ipsilateral lung is necessary to aid vision, this may not be possible if there is damage to the contralateral lung. This may be avoided by partial deflation with jet insufflation.
- Operator-dependent, with limited opportunities for developing expertise in most centres.
- Mini-thoracotomy may be required for therapeutic intervention.
- It is complicated or prevented by the presence of adhesions.

Further reading

Alexander-Williams J. Laparoscopy in abdominal trauma. *Injury,* 1994; **25:** 585–6.
McManus K, McGuigan J. Minimally invasive therapy in thoracic injury. *Injury,* 1994; **25:** 609–14.

Related topics of interest

LARYNGEAL FRACTURES

Fracture of the larynx is rare and generally results from direct trauma to the neck, commonly by impact with a steering wheel, penetrating trauma is a less common cause. A high index of suspicion is required.

Indications of laryngeal fracture

- Hoarseness or voice alteration.
- Swelling of the neck.
- Subcutaneous emphysema.
- Crepitus at the fracture site.
- Shortness of breath.
- Haemoptysis.

The initial management depends upon the degree of respiratory distress. In severe respiratory distress an attempt is made to pass an endotracheal tube: this should be performed by an expert. Failure to establish an airway in this manner warrants a cricothyroidotomy or formal tracheostomy.

Diagnosis is suggested by the presence of air in the soft tissues on a lateral and AP X-ray of the neck. Bronchoscopy will confirm the diagnosis and establish the site of injury. CT may also be of help in less severe cases.

Urgent referral to a thoracic or ENT surgeon is required for definitive management.

Related topics of interest

LOCAL BLOCKS: REGIONAL ANAESTHESIA

Regional anaesthesia ('blockade') is the use of local anaesthetic drugs to anaesthetize a region of the body, such as brachial plexus block for the upper limb. Regional techniques may be used alone for analgesia, or as a supplement to general anaesthesia.

Advantages
- Complete analgesia is possible which is rarely achievable with systemic drugs.
- No sedation, nausea, vomiting or respiratory depression.
- Possible limitation of stress response.
- May improve distal limb perfusion (sympathetic block).

Disadvantages
- Special training and skill needed.
- Significant failure rate.
- Onset may be delayed.
- Motor blockade.
- Risk of anaesthetic toxicity (see below).
- Masks neurological signs (may be contraindicated medico-legally in the presence of neurological deficit).
- Masks symptoms of compartment syndrome.

Local anaesthetic agents

Local anaesthetics block membrane depolarization in nerves and other excitable tissues. They are classed as:

1. *Esters.*

- Cocaine.
- Procaine.
- Benzocaine.
- Amethocaine.

2. *Amides.*

- Lignocaine.
- Prilocaine.
- Bupivacaine.
- Ropivacaine.

The most commonly used are:

- Lignocaine (0.5, 1 or 2% solution).
  - (a) Relatively rapid onset.
  - (b) Duration of effect 1–3 hours (prolonged by adrenaline).

- Prilocaine (0.5, 1 or 2% solution).
  (a) Relatively low potential for toxicity.
  (b) Similar onset and duration to lignocaine.
  (c) May cause methaemoglobinaemia.
- Bupivacaine (0.25 or 0.5% solutions).
  (a) Slower onset of effect; duration 3–16 hours (highly protein bound).
  (b) Potential for severe cardiotoxicity.

3. Concentration. Higher concentrations give a faster onset and more intense block, but lower volumes may be needed to keep within the toxic dose (see below).

4. Vasoconstrictors. By reducing systemic absorption, adrenaline-containing solutions usually have a more prolonged effect, and allow a higher dose of anaesthetic to be given. Never use near-end arteries (e.g. for digital nerve block).

5. Adverse effects.

- Toxicity (see below).
- Allergy: very rare, especially with amide drugs.
- Adrenaline effects: hypertension, tachycardia (use with caution in hypertension and ischaemic heart disease).

Local anaesthetic toxicity This arises from overdose, or intravascular injection. A membrane-stabilizing effect occurs in other excitable tissues (e.g. central nervous system and heart).

1. Features.

- Neurological: circumoral tingling, tinnitus, paraesthesia, drowsiness, coma, convulsions, apnoea.
- Cardiovascular: hypotension, bradycardia, arrhythmias.

2. Management.

- Discontinue the drug.
- Maintain the airway, give 100% oxygen, assist ventilation if necessary.
- Monitor blood pressure and ECG. Treat hypotension with a sympathomimetic (e.g. ephedrine). Avoid treating arrhythmias with lignocaine [bretylium is an alternative for ventricular fibrillation (VF)].

- Treat convulsions initially with IV diazepam.
- Consider ITU or high dependency unit (HDU) transfer.

3. Maximum safe doses.

- Lignocaine: 3 mg/kg (7 mg/kg with adrenaline).
- Prilocaine: 3 mg/kg for Biers block, otherwise 5 mg/kg (8 mg/kg with adrenaline).
- Bupivacaine: 2 mg/kg (3 mg/kg with adrenaline).

NB: an x% solution contains 10x mg/ml.

Principles of regional blockade

Choose the appropriate agent for example lignocaine or prilocaine for rapid onset; bupivicaine for a more prolonged effect.

- Do not exceed toxic dose.
- Use adrenaline only if appropriate (see above).
- Always aspirate before injection.
- Adjunctive sedation may be used, but will not compensate for an inadequate block.

For major regional blockade:

- Patients should be fasted as for general anaesthesia.
- Resuscitation facilities must be available.
- IV access is mandatory.
- ECG, blood pressure and pulse oximeter should be monitored.

Specific regional techniques

1. Biers block. Intravenous regional anaesthesia (IVRA). Injection of local anaesthetic into the veins of an isolated exsanguinated limb. Considered here in detail as it is commonly used, often by non-anaesthetists, and is potentially fatal if the drug enters the systemic circulation.

- Indications:
  (a) Forearm surgery and fracture reduction.
  (b) Occasionally for lower leg and foot surgery.
- Contraindications:
  (a) Sickle cell trait or anaemia.
  (b) Severe hypertension or peripheral vascular disease.
  (c) Local infection.
  (d) Children who would not tolerate a regional block.
- Preconditions:
  (a) Patients should be fasted as for general anaesthesia.

(b) Resuscitation facilities must be available.

(c) IVRA should only be performed by those with appropriate training.

(d) A doctor competent in resuscitation must be present throughout.

(e) IV access in opposite arm is essential.

- Technique: A vein on the dorsum of the affected hand is cannulated. After exsanguination, a reliable upper-arm tourniquet is inflated 100 mmHg above systolic BP. Prilocaine 0.5% 30–40 ml is injected slowly into this arm. (Bupivacaine is *not* used because of potential cardiac toxicity). The tourniquet is watched constantly, and kept at starting pressure throughout. After the procedure the tourniquet is deflated, but *not less than 20 min* after the original injection.

Other techniques

1. Brachial plexus block. Useful for surgery/analgesia of upper limb. Catheter techniques possible for prolonged analgesia or repeated surgery/dressings. Onset may be delayed (20–40 min). Types:

- Interscalene: most suitable for shoulder lesions, but ulnar block may be poor.
  Risks: epidural, intrathecal, or vertebral arterial injection, phrenic or recurrent laryngeal nerve palsy, Horner's syndrome
- Supraclavicular: this gives the most extensive limb block.
  Risks: pneumothorax (presentation may be delayed), subclavian arterial puncture, phrenic or recurrent laryngeal nerve palsy, Horner's syndrome.
- Axillary: the safest method, but not effective for shoulder/upper arm lesions. Musculocutaneous and axillary nerve block may be poor.

2. Digital nerve block. Suitable for finger and toe lesions. Effective and technically simple. Adrenaline-containing solutions should never be used.

3. Infiltration of a fracture haematoma. Sometimes used for reduction of wrist fractures, but not ideal.
  Risks: systemic infection, and also infection because a closed fracture has been converted into an open one.

4. *Intercostal block.* Suitable for rib fractures, flail chest, and anterior abdominal wall pain (T7 and below). There is relatively rapid systemic absorption.

> Risks: pneumothorax (avoid in presence of contralateral pneumothorax, and avoid bilateral blocks), local anaesthetic toxicity (limit number of nerve blocks).

5. *Femoral nerve block.* Suitable for fractured shaft of the femur, and lesions on the anterior thigh. Also suitable for lower leg lesions in combination with sciatic nerve block. Technically straightforward.

6 *Lateral cutaneous nerve of thigh block.* May be used together with femoral nerve block, for example for thigh skin grafts.

7. *3-in-1 block (femoral, obturator, and lateral cutaneous nerve of thigh).* Use an identical approach to femoral nerve block, with a larger volume of anaesthetic (spread up the fascial sheath).

> It is suitable for hip fractures/dislocations, and lesions of the medial, lateral and anterior thigh.

8. *Psoas compartment (lumbar plexus) block.* Suitable for hip/femoral neck fractures, and analgesia for most of lower limb (although sciatic block may be incomplete). It is technically difficult.

9. *Sciatic nerve block.* Gives anaesthesia of the back of the thigh, the anterolateral part of the leg, and most of the foot. It may be combined with femoral or 3-in-1 block for lesions of the thigh and leg (large volumes needed). Technically it is difficult.

Further reading

Illingworth KA, Simpson KH. *Anaesthesia and Analgesia in Emergency Medicine.* Oxford: Oxford University Press, 1994.
Wildsmith JAW, Armitage EN (eds). *Principles and Practice of Regional Anaesthesia,* 2nd Edn. Edinburgh: Churchill Livingstone, 1993.

Related topics of interest

LONG BONE FRACTURES

General considerations

Fracture patterns

The fracture pattern relates closely to the mechanism of injury. Direct trauma will produce a transverse fracture pattern (with or without comminution), often associated with gross soft-tissue involvement and destruction. Rotational forces tend to produce spiral fractures. Oblique fractures occur due to a combination of rotation, bending and loading, and may result in a *butterfly* fragment.

The possibility of a pathological fracture secondary to metastatic disease should always be considered, especially if the mechanism of injury appears inadequate to explain the fracture.

Fracture healing

If treated conservatively with external immobilization, the initial phase of tissue destruction and haematoma formation at the fracture site is followed by a phase of inflammation and cellular proliferation which leads to callus formation. This is followed by consolidation and remodelling. The micro-movements that occur with conservative management of fractures are thought to play a part in the generation of callus. This type of fracture healing does not occur with rigid internal fixation, when fracture healing depends on resorption of dead bone at the fracture ends with infiltration and healing across the fracture gap. Intramedullary fixation, which does not produce rigid fixation, is associated with callus formation.

Treatment

The following should be considered when selecting the most appropriate method of fracture treatment:

- Age.
- Likely physical demands.
- Fracture pattern.
- Whether the fracture is simple or compound.
- Degree of bony fragmentation and displacement.
- Joint involvement.

Long bone fractures may be managed by closed immobilization in plaster of Paris (or synthetic cast) with or without early mobilization in a functional cast, or by internal fixation. If an acceptable stable reduction cannot be achieved by closed methods, open reduction and fixation is mandatory.

Internal fixation aims to achieve a full and accurate reduction of the fracture and can be achieved in a number of ways, including intramedullary nailing (humerus, femur and tibia) and plating (radius and ulnar). Internal fixation is particularly appropriate in the patient with multiple injuries or the elderly patient in whom prolonged immobilization is associated with morbidity.

Most authorities would now accept that internal fixation is the treatment of choice for the majority of long bone fractures.

Open fractures

Previous apprehension regarding the treatment of open fractures by internal fixation has now been overcome. Combined management by orthopaedic and plastic surgeons is now recommended in severe open fractures. Initially, compound wounds should be covered with a Betadine®-soaked dressing while waiting for surgery. The open fracture is then converted into a closed fracture with internal or external fixation by the use of split skin grafting, fasciocutaneous and myofascial grafts as well as free flaps. This aggressive wound management is combined with adequate debridement and antibiotic cover.

Fractures of the shaft of the humerus

Fractures of the distal humerus are discussed in Elbow injuries, and of the proximal humerus in Shoulder injuries.

Mechanism of injury

These fractures usually result either from direct trauma or from a fall in which the humerus takes the force of the impact. A rotational element is usually present.

Clinical features

The arm is often held supported, and movements are painful. There is usually marked swelling, and often deformity. The radial nerve should be assessed routinely.

Radiology

Radiological confirmation of the site of the fracture will dictate the likely method of treatment.

Treatment

Shaft fractures heal well in a hanging cast followed by a functional brace. Unstable fractures can be treated by plating or intramedullary nail fixation.

Complications

Radial nerve palsy is common, in closed injuries this is usually due to a neuropraxia and 90% will recover spontaneously.

Fractures of the shafts of the radius and ulnar

Fractures of the radial head and neck, and of the olecranon are considered in Elbow injuries, and of the distal radius and ulnar in Wrist injuries.

Isolated radial fracture is associated with the risk of inferior radio-ulnar dislocation (*Galeazzi* fracture) and isolated ulnar fracture with superior radio-ulnar dislocation (*Monteggia* fracture).

Mechanism of injury	Commonly due to direct trauma or twisting forces. Monteggia and Galeazzi fractures follow a fall on an outstretched hand with associated rotation.
Clinical features	Pain, deformity and loss of function are common. In the case of radio-ulnar dislocation, bony prominence of the dislocated part may be found.
Radiology	The joint above and below any isolated fracture of a forearm bone must be visualized.
Treatment	Except in the case of the most minor single bone crack fractures, fractures of the shafts of the radius and ulnar are best treated by open reduction and internal fixation using plates.
Treatment of Monteggia and Galleazi fractures	These fractures are invariably treated in adults by open reduction and plating.
Complications	Except in the most minor cases, delayed union is relatively common with fractures of the radial and ulnar shafts (especially of the radius). Consideration should therefore be given to internal fixation which allows early mobilization and reduces the risk of this occurring.

Fractures of the shaft of the femur

Fractures of the femoral neck are considered in Hip fractures and dislocations.

Mechanism of injury	A great deal of force is required to fracture the shaft of a femur. Not surprisingly therefore, the most common mechanism of injury is direct trauma, usually from high-speed road-traffic accidents. Femoral shaft fractures commonly result from motorcyclists striking their thighs on the handlebars as they are thrown forwards off their bikes.

Clinical features	Marked deformity and angulation of the thigh may be present with significant swelling due to bleeding from the fracture. This bleeding may be cardiovascularly significant (particularly in bilateral or compound fractures) and should be controlled by direct pressure and appropriate splintage. The leg is commonly shortened and externally rotated. The foot may be noticed not to be pointing forward when the thigh is in the neutral position.
Radiology	Radiography will confirm the fracture as well as demonstrating the degree of comminution.
Treatment	The current treatment of choice is intramedullary nail fixation with distal and proximal locking, which maintains length and prevents relative rotation of the proximal and distal parts of the femur. Internal fixation allows earlier rehabilitation.
Complications	• Early: shock and fat embolism syndrome.
	• Intermediate: thromboembolism.
	• Late: delayed union, malunion and non-union. Infection following operative treatment.

Fractures of the tibia and fibula

Fractures of the distal tibia and fibula are considered in Ankle injuries: fractures.

Fractures of the tibial plateau

Mechanism of injury	Tibial plateau fractures usually result from varus or valgus forces when weight bearing as the femoral condyle damages the corresponding tibial plateau ('Bumper fracture').
Clinical features	The knee is swollen due to haemarthrosis and may be deformed.
Radiology	Radiographs will demonstrate the fracture, which should be defined, especially before surgery, by CT scanning.
Treatment	Except in undisplaced fractures and elderly patients, open reduction with buttress plating, and where necessary bone grafting, is the treatment of choice in order to restore the joint surface and permit early restoration of function.

| Complications | • Compartment syndrome. |
| | • Malunion and secondary osteoarthrosis. |

Fractures of the shafts of the tibia and fibula

Mechanism of injury	Complex fracture patterns occur in high-energy direct trauma, such as road-traffic accidents. Low-energy injuries produce variable fracture patterns, depending on whether there is an angulatory or rotational component to the force.
Clinical features	In open and closed fractures, the distal component of a fractured tibia is usually externally rotated. Associated neurovascular compromise may be noted.
Radiology	Will define the fracture pattern and must include clear views of the knee and ankle.
Treatment	Fractures of the tibia are best treated by intramedullary nailing with proximal and distal locking. This treatment is not contraindicated if the fracture is compound; however, in this situation it should follow wound debridement. In severe cases, consideration should be given to joint management with plastic surgeons.
	Isolated fibular shaft fractures are usually treated in a below-knee plaster or synthetic cast.
Complications	• Neurovascular injury.
	• Compartment syndrome.
	• Infection (compound fractures, or following surgery).
	• Delayed union, malunion or non-union.
	• Ankle and knee joint stiffness.

Long bone fractures in children

In children, fracture patterns are modified by the pliability of the bones and the presence of growth plates. Greenstick fractures are common. Most fractures are treated conservatively, with the exception of displaced fractures of both forearm bones when plate fixation may be necessary to prevent rotational deformity.

Further reading

Apley AG and Solomon L. *Apley's System of Orthopaedics and Fractures,* 7th Edn. Oxford: Butterworth Heinemann,1993.

Related topics of interest

MAXILLOFACIAL INJURIES

Oral and maxillofacial injuries are usually assessed during the secondary survey. Some injuries can be life threatening and must be managed during the primary survey and resuscitation phases.

Categories of injury

Injuries may be divided into:

1. *Soft tissue* (scalp and face).

2. *Hard tissue* (bone and teeth).

Maxillary fractures

- Mobile maxilla.
- Teeth not meeting properly (malocclusion).
- Bilateral facial swelling.
- Bilateral periorbital haematoma.

Mandibular fractures

- Mobile fragments of jaw.
- Teeth not meeting properly (malocclusion).
- Sublingual haematoma.
- Step deformity along lower border of jaw.

Life-threatening maxillofacial injuries are those which compromise the airway or cause uncontrollable haemorrhage.

Airway

1. *Displacement of the fractured maxilla.*

- Downward and backward displacement of the middle third of the facial skeleton along the inclined plane of the skull base.
   Disimpact by pulling maxilla forward.

2. *Loss of tongue control.*

- Bilateral fracture of the mandible allowing backward displacement of the anterior fragment by pull of the genioglossus muscle. This is particularly noticeable with a depressed level of consciousness.
   Pull tongue forward and hold using 0 gauge black silk or a large safety pin.

3. *Foreign bodies.*
- Teeth, dentures, bone fragments, vomitus or haematoma.

Finger sweep and suction (Yankauer design). Leave well-fitting and unbroken dentures in place. Exclude inhalation of lost teeth or fragments by chest X-ray. Avulsed teeth should be either immediately reinserted or carried in a suitable transport medium (e.g. milk).

4. *Haemorrhage.*

5. *Soft tissue swelling and oedema.*

• Occurs around the upper airway.
     The patient must be carefully monitored as the condition may gradually worsen over the following few hours.

6. *Direct trauma to the larynx and trachea.*

• Look for neck swelling, dyspnoea, and voice alteration.
     This type of trauma may need soft tissue X-rays of neck and mediastinum.

Cervical spine

Cervical spine injury occurs in 2% of maxillofacial trauma cases and must be excluded. The spine should be protected using a rigid collar and X-rays taken to show all the cervical vertebrae.

Haemorrhage control

Bleeding from the soft tissues of the face and scalp may be profuse due to the good blood supply to the area. Bony injuries may also be responsible for massive haemorrhage from the terminal branches of the maxillary artery and the anterior and posterior ethmoidal arteries.

1. *Complications:*

• Airway obstruction.
• Hypovolaemic shock.
(a) Open wounds.
     Assess wound for blood loss.
     Cover wound with gauze pack.
     Do not explore neck wounds in casualty – arteriography may be necessary.
(b) Closed wounds.
     Bleeding from nose and mouth.
     May need anterior and posterior nasal packs.

Use ribbon gauze anteriorly.

Use a 12/14 G Foley catheter and balloon posteriorly.

Nasal Epistats® used in conjunction with dental props provide tamponade in severe haemorrhage from fractures of the facial skeleton. Alternatively Merocel® expanding foam nasal packs may be used for rapid haemostasis.

Further reading

Dyer PV. Maxillofacial Trauma. In: Greaves I, Hodgetts T and Porter K (eds) *Emergency Care. A Textbook for Paramedics.* London: WB Saunders, 1997.

Hawksford J, Banks JG. *Maxillofacial and Dental Emergencies: Oxford Handbooks in Emergency Medicine.* Oxford: Oxford University Press, 1994.

Related topics of interest

Cervical spine injuries (p. 65)
Dental trauma (p. 76)
Head injuries (p. 124)
Laryngeal fractures (p. 183)
Ocular trauma (p. 212)

METABOLIC RESPONSE TO TRAUMA

A traumatic injury is any injury resulting from the external transfer of energy to the body (ranging from a road-traffic accident to an elective surgical procedure). Such injuries set into motion a complex series of, as yet, incompletely understood metabolic and circulatory changes designed to help the body cope with, and if survival occurs, recover from the injury. The response to trauma is best considered under two broad headings: metabolic changes and circulatory changes (see Shock).

Metabolic changes

These are traditionally divided into two phases:

* The ebb phase (early or low-flow phase).
* The flow phase (convalescent or high-flow phase).

The ebb phase

The ebb phase is characterized by a series of rapid responses to trauma designed to ensure the immediate survival of the animal by attenuating or, in mild trauma, abolishing the physiological effects of the injurious agent.

A fall in circulating volume causes centrally mediated autonomic stimulation of the adrenal medulla and release of catecholamines. The catecholamines have several important effects:

* Peripheral vasoconstriction.
* Central vasodilatation.
* Increased heart rate.
* Bronchiolar dilatation.
* Increased glycogenolysis in the liver.
* Inhibition of insulin release.
* Increased lipolysis in the adipose tissues.

These effects serve to maintain the circulation and oxygenation of the vital organs, and increase the availability of glucose for the anticipated increased metabolic demands. The importance of this adrenal response to trauma is readily seen in the poor resistance to trauma of the patient with adrenal suppression or failure and inadequate replacement therapy.

The patient will exhibit the classical clinical signs of peripheral shut down, cool, pale, clammy skin, increased depth and rate of respiration, tachycardia and possibly mild agitation.

In some cases the patient will experience a transient vasovagal syncopal episode. This is caused by cerebral hypoxia, secondary to hypotension due to peripheral arteriolar dilatation leading to pooling of blood. The patient is pale, cold and clammy and has a bradycardia. As the patient falls to the floor, cerebral circulation is restored and recovery is rapid.

Metabolic acidosis is a common finding in the ebb phase and is due to anaerobic metabolism secondary to tisue hypoperfusion.

The flow phase

Many victims of major trauma die early due to the inability of the body to compensate for the profound circulatory collapse that occurs. Those who survive the initial insult enter the flow phase. This is divided into two parts:

- The catabolic phase.
- The anabolic phase.

1. The catabolic phase

(a) Protein, glucose and fat metabolism. The hallmark of the catabolic phase is protein breakdown with a corresponding increase in urinary nitrogen excretion. Protein catabolism provides amino acid substrates (principally alanine) for gluconeogenesis in the liver. Lipolysis is inhibited, with a consequent preservation of adipose tissue at the expense of lean body mass.

(b) Sodium and water metabolism. Increased production of antidiuretic hormone (ADH) and aldosterone lead, respectively, to urinary water and sodium retention. Patients who have experienced relatively mild insults (e.g. elective surgical procedures) will require less than the expected sodium and water replacement in the first 24–48 hours, thereafter the basic daily requirement for those on IV fluids is approximately 150 mmol.

(c) Potassium metabolism. Potassium loss, secondary to protein breakdown, occurs during the catabolic phase. The basic daily requirement for those on IV fluids is approximately 60–80 mmol.

(d) Haematological changes:

- Thrombocytosis.
- Neutrophilia.
- Normochromic, normocytic anaemia.
- Sludging.

The increase in platelet count may reach levels of 1000 $\times 10^9$/l or more within the first few hours following injury.

Early mobilization or prophylaxis against venous thrombosis will reduce the risk of pulmonary embolism.

The neutrophil count also rises within the first few hours following injury and may reach levels of $30 \times 10^6/l$ or more. This neutrophilia is not due to infection, and antibiotics are not required except in the presence of clinical or microbiological evidence of infection.

The anaemia is due in the early phase to redistribution of fluid from the extracellular space, later to suppression of the bone marrow and haemoglobin synthesis and possibly also to red cell sludging.

Sludging is due to reduced flow in the capillary beds combined with the formation of large aggregates of red blood cells. Such sludging predisposes to cellular hypoxia, tissue infarction and venous thrombosis.

The catabolic phase may last for only a day or two in the case of minor trauma or minor elective surgery, or for many days or weeks in the case of major trauma, major surgery or in the presence of complications such as sepsis. Early aggressive resuscitation of major trauma combined with adequate analgesia and prompt management of complications will attenuate the catabolic phase.

2. *The anabolic phase.* Once the catabolic phase is over, the anabolic phase begins. Protein synthesis commences and is associated with an increase in insulin secretion and metabolic rate. The metabolic acidosis, characteristic of the ebb phase, is corrected with the return of aerobic metabolism. Tissue healing and build-up of muscle occur. The anabolic phase may continue for many months after apparent recovery from the initial insult has occurred.

Further reading

Walter JB, Talbot IC. *Walter and Israel's General Pathology,* 7th Edn. Edinburgh: Churchill Livingstone, 1996.

Related topics of interest

Adult respiratory distress syndrome (ARDS) (p. 7)
Shock (p. 26)

MISSED INJURIES

Certain injuries or complications of injuries have a reputation for being missed on initial presentation. This may be due to inexperience on the part of the doctor assessing the patient, failure to follow accepted practices of examination or investigation or as a consequence of some specific feature of the injury which makes it prone to being missed. This is a summary of the most important of these injuries.

Bony injuries

As well as difficulty in assessing the patient because of age or mental status and inadequate examination, fractures may be missed because:

- Radiography was not requested because of failure to suspect a fracture based upon the clinical findings.
- The wrong side was X-rayed because of an error in clinical examination or use of abbreviations on the request form.
- The wrong radiographs were taken because of inadequate history on the request form (e.g. suspecting a scaphoid fracture and requesting a wrist radiograph with no mention of the suspicion of the scaphoid injury).
- Inadequate views were obtained (e.g. failure to obtain a view from C1–T1 on a lateral cervical spine view).
- Failure to interpret the radiograph correctly (e.g. attributing a skull fracture to a vascular marking or suture).

Therefore when requesting radiography, always take a history and perform a complete physical examination before filling in the request form. On the request form request the appropriate views, writing the side of the suspected lesion in full, not using abbreviations (e.g. RIGHT not R).

When reviewing the radiographs always ensure that the name on the films corresponds to the patient's name, and that correct and adequate views have been obtained and that the side radiographed corresponds with the side of the suspected lesion.

It is important to be conversant with the normal radiographic anatomy of the region in question and to know the common variants likely to be encountered. If in doubt, obtain a second, more experienced opinion.

Cervical spine injury

As mentioned above, cervical spine injury may be missed because of failure to obtain a complete series of cervical spine views with adequate exposure from C1 to T1. In the unconscious trauma victim, hypotension in the presence of a relative bradycardia may be an early sign of cervical cord lesion. This may initially be attributed to hypovolaemic shock; failure to respond to a fluid challenge should arouse suspicion.

Although the forces required to cause a fracture of the odontoid are usually considerable, in the elderly or very young such injuries may occur in association with suprisingly mild trauma.

A high index of suspicion of the possibility of cervical spine injury in any injury above the clavicle or in a deceleration-type injury is required. A thorough neurological assessment and examination to exclude local signs of injuries combined with normal cervical spine views (AP, lateral and oclontoid peg view) will exclude the majority of cervical spine injuries. If any doubt exists as to the possibility of such an injury, particularly in the elderly or young, further views under expert supervision with CT and/or MRI scans may be required.

Spinal cord injury without radiological abnormality (SCIWORA) may account for up to 50% of cervical cord injuries in children. A full neurological examination in a co-operative patient is required to exclude this injury. This examination may have to be delayed in a patient who is initially unconscious.

Posterior dislocation of the shoulder

The diagnosis of anterior dislocation of the shoulder rarely presents any great difficulty. Posterior dislocations, on the other hand, are notorious for presenting late. The incidence of posterior to anterior dislocations is approximately 50 : 1. there are two main reasons for this injury being missed:

1. Failure to interpret the radiographs correctly/failure to request adequate views. If the diagnosis is not suspected, only an AP view may be taken. On such a view the humeral head appears to be in correct anatomical alignment with the glenoid and the dislocation may be missed. In fact on such a view the head of the humerus will look abnormal (like an electric-light bulb). A lateral view will clearly show the posterior dislocation.

2. Failure to suspect the injury. Posterior dislocations are associated with victims of epileptic fits or electric shock. The injury will be missed in the initial phase because the patient is unconscious. Failure to adequately assess the patient prior to discharge and suspect the lesion, despite complaints of shoulder pain, compound the initial error.

Monteggia and Galeazzi fractures/dislocations

The *Monteggia* fracture dislocation is a fracture of the ulna associated with dislocation of the radial head at the proximal radio-ulnar joint and results from a fall on to the outstretched hand. The *Galeazzi* fracture dislocation is a fracture of the shaft of the radius associated with dislocation of the distal ulna.

Although the fractures are unlikely to be missed, the dislocations may be missed due to failure to obtain views of the whole forearm including both proximal and distal radio-ulnar joints. In the presence of a single forearm fracture, the possibility of a Monteggia or Galeazzi fracture dislocation should be considered and excluded. Adequate views should be obtained, including AP and true lateral views.

Scaphoid fracture

This fracture is probably not as commonly missed as in previous times, due to the wide publicity given to this missed injury (mainly in the medical defence agencies press!). Fracture of the scaphoid is missed because of inexperience and failure to recognize the presentation and appropriate management of this injury.

The notorious reputation of poor outcome from missed scaphoid fracture is attributable to the anomalous blood supply to the bone in certain individuals. The blood supply to the scaphoid is by a series of small blood vessels which enter the bone via the oblique ridge running between the two articular surfaces. In 30% of people the vessels enter at the distal part of ridge only. In this group of patients fractures of the waist or proximal pole result in ischaemia of the bone proximal to the fracture, with a consequent risk of avascular necrosis (complicating 30% of proximal pole fractures).

Because of the tight packing of bones in the carpus, a fracture line may not be visible for 10–14 days, at which time resorption of bone will leave a characteristic line.

Scaphoid fracture should be expected in anybody with tenderness in the anatomical snuffbox after injury. Additional signs include discomfort on axial compression of the thumb and tenderness over the dorsum of the scaphoid. If no fracture is evident on the initial films, the arm should be placed in a scaphoid plaster for 12–14 days. After this time the plaster is removed and the limb re-examined for any evidence of scaphoid tenderness. Such tenderness should lead to repeat views being requested and comparison with the old views for evidence of a fracture (the precise management of radiologically negative scpahoid injuries will vary from centre to centre, this protocol is one commonly used system).

Lunate dislocation

The most common carpal dislocation, this injury is frequently missed despite the considerable pain and swelling it causes, because of failure to interpret the radiographs correctly.

The injury is best seen on the lateral view of the wrist when the normal alignment of the lunate with the capitate (the capitate sits in the cup of the lunate) is lost, with the crescent shape of the lunate being made clear. On the AP view the normal square profile of the lunate, lying lateral to the scaphoid, becomes shaped like a processed cheese segment. The joint space between the lunate and scaphoid becomes obliterated and the lunate may appear to partially overlie the scaphoid.

Lunate dislocations may be associated with median nerve compression.

Maissoneuve fracture

This is a fracture of the proximal fibula, with diastasis (separation) of the distal talofibular joint and subluxation of the talus. The significant component of this fracture is the subluxation of the talus.

This injury is missed because of the failure to realize that an isolated fibula fracture above the inferior talofibular joint must be associated with a diastasis. The ankle is usually radiographed in isolation as this is the major area of pain. The finding of an isolated transverse medial malleolar fracture on ankle views should raise the possibility of such an injury and should lead to the request for full views of the tibia and fibula and examination of the ankle mortice; stress films may be required.

Soft-tissue injuries

Achilles tendon rupture

The patient presents with a history of undertaking strenuous exercise (e.g. squash) and feeling as if someone has kicked them in the back of the heel. The Achilles tendon may be partially or completely ruptured. Partial rupture may be difficult to exclude and may present later as a complete rupture. Clinical suspicion may be confirmed by ultrasound.

Complete rupture, if suspected, can be easily diagnosed. There may be a characteristic hollow over the tendon when compared with the normal side, although this is not always evident. The tiptoe test, where the patient demonstrates weakness of plantar flexion when asked to stand on tiptoes is not invariably abnormal and should not be relied on.

The most reliable test is *Simmond's* test. The patient is placed prone with the feet overhanging the edge of the examination couch and the calf squeezed. If the tendon is intact the foot plantarflexes, if the tendon is ruptured the foot does not move. This test will not demonstrate a partial rupture.

Complete rotator cuff tears

This is usually a complication of a fall on to the outstretched hand or while undertaking strenuous exercise (e.g. weightlifting). There is severe pain and localized tenderness over the deltoid with restricted movement and loss of abduction due to rupture of the supraspinatus tendon. The loss of abduction may be attributed to pain. The injury is often diagnosed as a 'sprain'.

In the acute phase the injury may be suspected as a result of the mechanism of injury and obvious loss of abduction: passive abduction may be limited and painful. Injection of local anaesthetic into the painful area will allow a partial tear to be diagnosed by the return of abduction and a complete tear to be diagnosed by loss of abduction below 90°, but maintenance of the arm in abduction above 90°, by the action of the deltoid.

Complete quadriceps tendon rupture

Following an injury in which extension at the knee is opposed, either the suprapatellar or infrapatellar portion of the quadriceps tendon may rupture. The patient will complain of pain at the site of the injury and difficulty in walking.

This injury is missed because of failure specifically to examine the quadriceps mechanism. The patient is laid supine and asked to straight leg raise against gravity, failure to do so indicates disruption of the quadriceps mechanism, a gap in the tendon at the site of rupture may be felt. In the presence of a partial tear of the quadriceps muscle, straight leg raising may be restricted due to pain, administration of a NSAID relieves the pain and allows the test to be performed.

The following soft tissue injuries are also frequently missed and are covered in other key topics:

- Compartment syndrome.
- Nerve injuries.
- Tendon injuries (see Hand injuries).
- Degloving injuries (see Soft-tissue injuries).

Further reading

Apley AG, Solomon L. *Apley's System of Orthopaedics and Fractures*, 7th Edn. Oxford: Butterworth Heinemann, 1993.

McRae R. *Practical Fracture Treatment,* 3rd Edn. Edinburgh: Churchill Livingstone, 1994.

Unwin A, Jones K. *Emergency Orthopaedics and Trauma.* Oxford: Butterworth Heinemann, 1995.

Related topics of interest

NAILBED INJURIES

Nailbed injuries are common within the A&E setting. Adequately managed they give rise to few long-term cosmetic or functional problems. Despite this the management of such injuries gives rise to much controversy.

Nailbed injuries occur most frequently in the 1–3 year age group and predominately in males. They are commonly caused by trapping a finger or fingers in the hinge end of a door. In this age group less than 10% will have a significant fracture to the terminal phalanx.

Treatment

There is debate as to whether all such injuries require nail removal to inspect the nailbed for damage. Generally the presence of a large subungual haematoma, deformity of the nail or displaced fracture of the terminal phalanx indicate that exploration of the nailbed is required.

Displaced laceration to the nailbed or laceration of the germinal matrix require repair to avoid future nail deformity. The nailbed itself is difficult to suture because of the underlying bone. It is usually sufficient to replace the viable parts of the nailbed and suture the lateral nailfold margins and/or the skin at the tip of the nailbed reshaping the bed back to its normal position using synthetic non-absorbable monofilament. Lacerations to the germinal matrix should be accurately approximated with a small (5/0 or 6/0 synthetic non-absorbable monofilament). Failure to correct the germinal matrix accurately may result in a deformed nail.

Displaced fractures of the terminal phalanx will be corrected by accurate suturing of the soft tissues. Practices vary with regard to the use of prophylactic antibiotics. One school of thought is that all nailbed injures associated with a fractured terminal phalanx require antibiotic cover. Many manage such injuries successfully by adequate wound cleansing and follow-up.

Sutures can generally be removed at 5 days, patients should be warned that even after correct management nail deformities can occur.

The fate of the removed or avulsed nail is controversial. Some replace the nail into the nailbed, claiming that it 'splints' the nailbed and prevents adhesions forming in the germinal matrix. Others discard the nail and apply a simple dressing to the nailbed. There is no evidence to support the superiority of either method and the choice is a matter of personal preference.

Further reading

Wilson GR, Nee PA, Watson JS. *Emergency Management of Hand Injuries*. Oxford Handbooks of Emergency Medicine. Oxford: Oxford University Press, 1997.

Related topic of interest

NON-ACCIDENTAL INJURY TO CHILDREN (NAI)

Non-accidental injury is a form of child abuse characterized by physical abuse. The definition is not absolute, but must be put in the context of the culture in which the child lives. Physical abuse may be active in that the child is directly injured by the carer, or passive by failure to maintain a safe environment or to provide adequate supervision.

Epidemiology

It is estimated that 100 children die every year in Britain as a direct result of physical abuse, although the true figure is undoubtedly higher. For every death there are many more children who suffer permanent disability as a result of their abuse.

Risk factors

The following are known to be associated with increased risk of a child being physically abused, the absence of one or all of these factors does not exclude the possibility of abuse.

- Birth weight < 2500 g.
- Mother aged < 30 years.
- Unwanted pregnancy.
- Marital stress.
- Lower socio-economic class.

Diagnosis

The mainstay of diagnosis is the suspicion that abuse may have occurred in the first place. The following features may suggest (but do not necessarily prove) that abuse has taken place.

- Inappropriate delay in seeking medical advice.
- Failure to seek medical advice.
- The history of the injury is vague or inconsistent.
- The history of the injury is not consistent with the injury.
- The parents' reaction is inappropriate.
  - (a) Lack of concern for the child's condition.
  - (b) Hostility to questions.
  - (c) Attempt to leave before the examination or treatment is completed.
- The child reacts inappropriately to its parents.
- There is a failure to thrive.
- The child volunteers that the parent or carer caused the injury.

- The presence of frozen watchfulness (uncommon).
- Previous injuries to the child or a sibling.

Characteristic patterns of injury

Although any injury may be caused by physical abuse, several patterns of injury are recognized as being associated with non-accidental injury:

- Bruising to the face.
- Finger shaped bruising, particularly bruises the size of adult fingers.
- Linear bruises.
- Burns, particularly cigarette burns.
- Abrasions.
- Different aged bruises (although such a pattern on the shins is common in non-abuse children).
- Subconjunctival haemorrhages.
- Retinal haemorrhages.
- Hyphaema.
- Bulging fontanelle.
- Adult human bite marks.
- Torn frenulum (not pathognomonic).

Bruising

Assessing the age of a bruise is notoriously difficult. Factors determining the presence and appearance of a bruise include:

- The child's skin colour.
- The blood supply to the injured area (bruises on the external ear appear later than bruises in more vascular areas).
- The depth of the bruise (bruises to the thigh may take several days to appear or may not appear at all at the site of injury and be inferred only by the secondary dependent bruising appearing days after the injury).

In general only two broad ages of bruise can be identified with any degree of intra-observer agreement.

1. *Red*   < 24 hours.

2. *Yellow*   > 48 hours.

Radiological features of non-accidental injury

- Any fracture in a child under 3 years (94% of fractures in abused children occur in the under threes).

- Metaphyseal flake fractures of the long bones.
- Spiral fractures of the long bones in infants.
- Fractures with epiphyseal displacement.
- Multiple rib fractures on chest X-ray.
- Multiple fractures of different ages on skeletal survey.
- Healing fractures suggesting inappropriate delay in seeking medical help.

NB: clavicular fracture and toddlers fractures may commonly present late.

Management

The immediate focus is to prevent further injury to the child. Any child suspected of being a victim of child abuse should be referred to the on-call paediatrician. The parents should not be confronted nor should accusations be made at this stage. The decision as to further investigations (including skeletal survey) rests with the paediatrician. Careful notes should be kept including verbatim accounts of the circumstances and timing of the injury. Charts are useful for recording the anatomical location and dimensions of other injuries. Photographs are invaluable, but should probably be deferred until the lead clinician assessing the patient had been involved.

If parents attempt to remove the child from hospital or refuse admission then two emergency procedures to prevent removal can be instituted:

- The police have the power to take a child into police protection.
- The social services department may undertake to obtain an emergency protection order allowing the child to be admitted to hospital for 8 days.

Further reading

Glasgow JFT and Graham HK. *Management of Injuries in Children.* London: BMJ Publishing Group, 1997.
Meadow R. *ABC of Child Abuse,* 2nd Edn. London: BMJ Publishing Group, 1993.

Related topic of interest

Paediatric aspects of trauma (p. 216)

OCULAR TRAUMA

Significant ocular trauma requires expert help. Early intervention before such help arrives will reduce the likelihood of further damage and may increase the probability of saving the sight in the affected eye.

History

1. *Ophthalmic.*

- Pre-existing eye disease.
- Use of contact lenses.
- Use of topical drugs to the eye.

2. *The mechanism of injury.*

- Blunt, penetrating, blast or flash.
- The presence of broken glass.
- The presence of chemical agents.

3. *The initial presenting complaint.*

- Pain.
- Foreign body sensation.
- Photophobia.

If the vision is impaired assess:

- The degree of impairment.
- Time after injury of onset of impairment.
- Progression of such impairment (i.e. immediate loss of vision or progressive loss of vision).

Examination

Following the taking of the history a detailed systematic examination of the eye should be made in an 'outside in' manner. The following should be examined:

1. *Visual acuity.*

- Snellen chart (may not be possible initially).
- Ability to count fingers.
- Ability to distinguish light and dark.
- Diplopia (may indicate orbital floor fracture).

2. *Eyelids.* These should be examined for the presence of:

- Swelling.
- Bruising.
- Lacerations.

- Burns.
- Ptosis.
- Subtarsal foreign bodies.

Indications for referral to an ophthalmic surgeon include lacerations involving:

- Lid margins.
- Levator muscle.
- Tear glands.
- Tear ducts.

Penetrating foreign bodies should likewise be referred, they should not be removed prior to referral.

3. *Orbital margins.* Palpate for:

- A 'step-off' deformity indicating a rim fracture.
- Subcutaneous emphysema suggesting a fracture into the ethmoid air sinus medially or the maxillary antrum inferiorly.

4. *Globe.* Examine for:

- Proptosis suggesting a retrobulbar haematoma (requiring urgent drainage to preserve sight).
- Posterior or inferior displacement suggesting orbital fracture.
- Elution of fluorescein during corneal examination suggesting penetrating injury to the globe. A ruptured globe should be gently padded, avoiding pressure, and ophthalmic advice sought.

5. *Pupils.* Examine for:

- Shape.
- Size.
- Regularity.
- Equality.
- Reactivity.

6. *Cornea.* Examine for:

- Corneal opacity.
- Abrasions (using fluorescein and a blue light).
- Foreign bodies. Small foreign bodies can be visualized with the aid of magnification. Superficial foreign bodies can be removed using topical anaesthetic.

Embedded foreign bodies and rust rings require ophthalmic intervention.

7. *Conjunctiva.* Examine for:

- Chemosis.
- Subconjunctival haemorrhage.
- Superficial foreign bodies.
- Subhyaloid haemorrhage or scleral haemorrhage without a posterior margin (suggesting basal skull fracture).
- Subconjunctival emphysema (suggesting fracture of the orbit into the ethmoid sinus or maxillary antrum).

8. *Anterior chamber.* Examine for:

- Hyphaema (the presence of blood in the anterior chamber) in its early stages this may not present as a fluid level and may appear as clouding of the anterior chamber on ophthalmoscopy.
- Shallow anterior chamber suggesting an anterior penetrating wound.
- Deep anterior chamber suggesting a posterior penetrating wound.

9. *Iris.* The iris should be round, regular and reactive to light. Any abnormality suggests a tear.

10. *Lens.* Examine for:

- Clarity.
- Position (the lens may be displaced or partially dislocated either anteriorly or posteriorly).

11. *Vitreous.* Examine for:

- Intraocular foreign body.
- Vitreous haemorrhage: this produces a dark rather than a red-light reflex).

12. *Retina.* Examine for:

- Tears.
- Detachment.
- Haemorrhage.

Chemical injuries   These should be treated by copious irrigation with normal saline or Hartmann's solution following application of topical local anaesthetic. Acid burns tend to be more superficial than alkali burns. Neutralizing agents should not be used as the heat generated by their chemical reaction can exacerbate existing damage.

Further reading

American College of Surgeons Committee on Trauma. Abdominal trauma. In: *Advanced Trauma Life Support: Program for Physicians*. Chicago: American College of Surgeons, 1993; 141–58.
Skinner D, Driscoll P, Earlam R. *ABC of Major Trauma*. London: BMJ Publications, 1991; 46–50.

Related topics of interest

Brainstem death and organ transplantation (p. 50)
Head injuries (p. 124)
Maxillofacial injuries (p. 195)

PAEDIATRIC ASPECTS OF TRAUMA

Trauma is the most common cause of death in children between the ages of 1 and 16 years in the developed world. This predominance of trauma deaths continues until well into the fourth decade of life. Traumatic death accounts for approximately 500 childhood deaths per year in the UK.

Epidemiology

1. Distribution. The pattern of trauma deaths in children follows the trimodal distribution described by Trunkey:

- Immediate deaths: death resulting from unsurvivable or effectively unsurvivable injury. Such deaths commonly occur at the scene or shortly after arrival at hospital. Little in the way of modern medical technology can contribute to prevention of the majority of such deaths. The only hope of reducing the burden of these deaths lies in the fields of public health, engineering and legislation.
- Early deaths: deaths resulting from airway obstruction, breathing problems, circulatory insufficiency and neurological injury. The majority of such deaths have been shown to be preventable with early access to hospital, early aggressive resuscitation and, where appropriate, prompt, appropriate, expert surgery.
- Late deaths: death resulting from, in the majority of cases, multisystem failure or sepsis. These deaths often occur on the intensive care unit. A proportion of such deaths may be prevented by adequate early management as outlined above.

It should be noted that Trunkey described his distribution of deaths based upon mode of death. This is often misquoted as time of death (<1 hour, 1–4 hours and more than 4 hours). This error is a result of misreading his original article and has led to confusion as to the relative proportion of deaths occurring in each modality in different studies.

2. Incidence. For the purposes of trauma audit, major trauma is defined as injury resulting in an Injury Severity Score (ISS) of 16 or over, an injury resulting in death or an injury resulting in admission to an ITU.

Penetrating major trauma is exceptionally uncommon in children in the UK, one study reporting no cases of penetrating trauma in a single region in one year. The incidence of blunt trauma in children is approximately 10% that of adults, resulting in an incidence of blunt trauma in children arriving alive at hospital of approximately 1:10 000 new A&E attenders (adult incidence approximately 1:1000). The average District General Hospital may therefore expect to see only 5–10 cases of paediatric major trauma per year.

Of blunt major trauma, approximately one-third are isolated head injuries, one-third are extremity or torso injuries and one-third are a combination of head injuries and extremity or torso injuries.

Early management of paediatric trauma

The initial management priorities for paediatric trauma are the same as for adult trauma:

- **A**irway control with cervical spine immobilization.
- **B**reathing.
- **C**irculation and haemorrhage control.
- **D**isability (neurological assessment).
- **E**xposure and environmental control.

Problems identified during this initial phase of resuscitation (the primary survey) should be addressed immediately before proceeding on to the next step of the assessment.

Children are particularly prone to hypoglycaemia, and a rapid estimation of blood glucose using one of the reagent sticks should be made early on in the initial resuscitation. If hypoglycaemia is present, it should be corrected with an initial dose of 5 ml/kg of 10% glucose (stronger solutions are not recommended as they may result in cerebral oedema). The response to this dose should be assessed and further aliquots given as required. This glucose volume should be given in addition to any volume replacement estimates for shock.

Resuscitating the injured child

It is a commonly quoted and true adage that children *are not just little adults*. There are a number of differences between adults and children which must be taken into account during trauma resuscitation and subsequently.

1. General considerations.

- Size: children's physical dimensions vary both within and between age groups. Easy availability of a reference chart (or Broselow tape) will aid in determining the correct dosage of drugs for each child. Such charts give an estimate of weight based upon the child's age and length (such estimates are based upon the fiftieth centile values for male children).

- Weight: a simple formula relating age to weight in the over-one age group is:

$$\text{Weight (kg)} = 2 \times (\text{age} + 4).$$

- Body proportions: the surface area to volume ratio varies with age, being at its maximum in the infant. The immediate consequence of this is that children lose heat at a faster rate than adults and are more likely to suffer hypothermia if left uncovered for prolonged periods during resuscitation. Similarly, the relative proportions of different body parts vary with age. In the burned child specific charts are available for calculation of the burn area, taking into account the variation in relative body proportion with age.

2. *Specific features.* The following features of the child's anatomy pose potential airway problems when conscious level is impaired:

(a) larger head and shorter neck, leading to neck flexion;
(b) larger tongue;
(c) compressible floor of mouth;
(d) loose primary dentition;
(e) adenotonsillar hypertrophy.

In addition the large tongue, the horseshoe-shaped epiglottis and the high anterior larynx all combine to make intubation more difficult for the inexperienced. If the child is to be intubated, the correct tube size may be estimated by reference to a standard chart. If no chart is available, the tube size may be approximated to the diameter of the *child's* little finger or nostril. Alternately the following formula can be used:

$$\text{Tube diameter} = \text{age}/4 + 4.$$

- Cervical spine injury is uncommon in children, but devastating if missed. All children who have suffered major trauma or have an appropriate mechanism of injury should be suspected of having a spinal injury until proven otherwise. Immobilization of the cervical spine with a semi-rigid collar, sandbags and tape, or collar and paediatric long spinal board should be carried out. Cervical cord injury can occur in the absence of vertebral injury, there may not therefore be any radiological evidence of such injury. In all cases where there is a strong suspicion of such an injury the cervical spine should remain immobilized until cleared by an experienced doctor. In the child (unlike the adult), the majority of bony cervical spine injuries occur in the upper cervical spine.

The use of long spinal boards is now common. Originally intended as a extrication and transport device, they are now used during the early phase of resuscitation for cervical spine immobilization. Children should be kept on such boards for the minimum period of time. If a child is agitated and unco-operative, it is best not to use sandbags and tape. These will only serve to immobilize the cervical spine against a moving body and may exacerbate any cord injury. In such circumstances the child should be left in a semi-rigid collar with manual immobilization if tolerated, or manual immobilization alone while urgent radiographs are completed. Sedation, paralysis and intubation may be necessary, depending on the associated injuries.

- Breathing: the compliant chest wall of the child tends to deform more under stress than an adult's, leading to the possibility of significant damage to the underlying lung even in the absence of rib fracture.
- The child's circulating blood volume (80 ml/kg) is greater per kilogram body weight than the adult's. Children have a greater capacity to compensate for circulating volume loss than adults and may be significantly hypovolaemic before clear clinical signs of shock are evident. However, at the end of the compensatory phase decompensation is rapid and catastrophic, early aggressive fluid resuscitation in the presence of signs of circulatory impairment is therefore imperative. Signs of potential or actual circulatory failure include:
  (a) mental impairment;
  (b) cold peripheries;
  (c) absent or weak peripheral pulses;
  (d) pale or mottled extremities;
  (e) delayed capillary refill.

The normal physiological ranges for the commonly measured parameters (BP, pulse, respiratory rate) vary with age and are available on standard reference charts. A simple formula for estimating the fifth centile value for systolic pressure in the over one age group is:

$$\text{Fifth centile systolic BP} = 70 + (\text{age} \times 2).$$

A value below this level indicates that decompensated shock is present and that urgent, aggressive fluid resuscitation is required. The initial fluid resuscitation bolus should be 20 ml/kg of colloid or crystalloid (normal saline or Hartmann's solution, not dextrose-containing fluids). This bolus should be followed by a clinical assessment of the response and further boluses as required. Any child requiring more than 40 ml/kg resuscitation requires blood and a surgical assessment.

Normal values of commonly measured parameters in the child

Age (years)	Respiratory rate (breaths/min)	Pulse rate (beats/min)	Systolic blood pressure (mmHg)
Newborn	–	160	60–80
<1	30–40	110–160	70–90
1–5	25–30	95–140	80–100
6–12	20–25	80–120	90–110
13+	–	60–100	100–120

- Disability (neurological assessment): during the initial phase a formal assessment of conscious level using the Glasgow Coma Score is not required, the AVPU scale along with an assessment of pupillary size and response provides sufficient information on which to base management decisions:

A Alert
V Responds to voice
P Responds to pain
U Unresponsive

- Full assessment requires removal of the child's clothes. As mentioned above, this should be done only to the extent, and for the minimum time, required, so as to reduce heat loss and save embarrassment.

Non-accidental injury   Major trauma in any child under the age of one should raise the strong suspicion of the possibility of non-accidental injury.

Further reading

Advanced Life Support Group. *Advanced Paediatric Life Support: The Practical Approach.* London: BMJ Publishing Group, 1993.

American College of Surgeons Committee on Trauma. Advanced Trauma Life Support Course, 1993.

Glasgow JFT, Graham HK. *Management of Injuries in Children.* London: BMJ Publishing Group, 1997.

Morton RJ, Phillips BM. *Accidents and Emergencies in Children*, 2nd Edn. Oxford: Oxford University Press, 1996.

Related topics of interest

Advanced Trauma Life Support (ATLS) (p. 11)
Non-accidental injury to children (NAI) (p. 209)

PATHOLOGICAL FRACTURES

A pathological fracture is a fracture through an area of bone weakened by disease. Such fractures may occur after apparently trivial injuries, or may occur spontaneously. The fracture may be the initial presentation of the underlying pathological condition.

Causes of pathological fractures

1. Generalized bone disease.

- Osteogenesis imperfecta.
- Osteoporosis.
- Metabolic/endocrine bone disease
    - hyperparathyroidism
    - osteomalacia
    - vitamin C deficiency
    - Cushing's disease
    - hyperthyroidism.
- Osteopetrosis.
- Neurofibromatosis.
- Gaucher's disease.
- Enchondromatosis.
- Myelomatosis.
- Polyostic fibrous dysplasia.
- Paget's disease.

2. Local benign conditions.

- Chronic infection.
- Solitary bone cyst.
- Fibrous cortical defect.
- Chondromyxoid fibroma.
- Aneurysmal bone cyst.
- Chondroma.
- Monostotic fibrous dysplasia.

3. Primary malignant bone tumours.

- Chondrosarcoma.
- Osteosarcoma.
- Ewing's tumour.

4. Metastatic tumours.

- Breast.
- Lung.
- Bowel.

	• Kidney.
	• Thyroid.
	• Prostate.

Investigation   In the majority of cases the history and examination, in combination with the patient's age and sex, will suggest the diagnosis. Plain radiographs of the fracture will suggest the possibility of local disease (e.g. bone cyst or metastasis) or more generalized disease (e.g. osteoporosis).

Other investigations will be suggested by the clinical findings and may include the following:

- Full blood count.
- Erythrocyte sedimentation rate.
- Protein electrophoresis.
- Urine for Bence Jones protein and electrophoretic strip.
- Isotope bone scan.
- Chest radiograph.
- Bone biopsy if indicated.

Treatment   In the majority of cases of generalized bone disease and malignant disease internal fixation is the method of choice. In the case of localized benign disease the fracture may be treated as for a normal fracture at that site.

Further reading

Apley AG, Solomon L. *Apley's System of Orthopaedics and Fractures*, 7th Edn. Oxford: Butterworth Heinemann, 1993.

Related topics of interest

Hip fractures and dislocations (p. 138)
Long bone fractures (p. 189)

PELVIC FRACTURES

Pelvic fractures may range from critical life-threatening injuries to relatively trivial injuries causing nothing more than discomfort. Significant pelvic fractures are the result of transfers of large amounts of energy and are commonly associated, therefore, with other serious injuries. These injuries may be divided into injuries to structures around the pelvis (bladder, gut and reproductive organs) and injuries to structures not directly associated with the pelvis (chest and head injuries).

Emergency assessment

The emergency management of pelvic fractures follows conventional ATLS protocols. A careful physical examination must include examination of the urethral opening and a rectal examination to exclude the penetration of these organs by bony pelvic fragments. If significant pubic rami fractures are demonstrated on radiography or there is vaginal bleeding, a vaginal examination will also be necessary. Pelvic injuries may need to be considered at an early stage of resuscitation if the pelvis fracture is associated with major haemorrhage. This is particularly likely to be the case in high-energy trauma resulting in a significant degree of displacement of fragments or significant opening of the pelvic ring.

Major haemorrhage is normally predominantly venous, and occurs not only because of soft-tissue damage but also because disruption of the pelvis produces a larger diameter ring into which bleeding can continue without significant tamponade.

Prompt restoration of the pelvic diameter, therefore, is the most important factor in control of severe haemorrhage. External fixation may therefore be necessary in the resuscitation room. Embolization of bleeding pelvic vessels is becoming used increasingly in these situations. Temporizing measures include the application of a MAST suit or extrication device.

Classification of pelvic fractures

Although complex classification systems exist to define the morphology of pelvic fractures, broadly speaking, these fractures may be classified into three groups:

- Fractures not involving the integrity of the pelvic ring.
- Fractures involving the integrity of the pelvic ring.
- Fractures involving the acetabulum.

Fractures not involving the integrity of the pelvic ring

These fractures include fractures of the wing of the ilium, avulsion fractures associated with muscle origins and fractures of a single pubic ramus.

1.   Fractures of the wing of the ilium. The wing of the ilium is fractured by direct trauma or crushing injuries. Blood loss may be considerable due to the bone's muscle coverage. Bruising from damage to the glutei may be marked.

Pain usually settles over a few days, following which mobilization can be started. Markedly displaced fractures may need reduction and internal fixation.

2.   Avulsion fractures associated with muscle origins. These fractures occur most commonly in athletes after sudden muscular contraction:

- Anterior inferior spine – rectus femoris.
- Ischial tuberosity – hamstrings.
- Posterior spine – erector spinae.
- Crest of ilium – abdominal muscles.

In these cases, rest and symptomatic treatment are generally all that is required; however, in high-performance athletes, surgical intervention and fixation should be considered.

3.   Fractures of a single pubic ramus. These fractures usually occur in the elderly following relatively minor trauma. Fracture of a single ramus is rare. Treatment is mobilization following a short period of bed rest.

Fractures involving the integrity of the pelvic ring

These fractures may be subclassified according to mechanism of injury:

1.   Lateral compression fractures. A sideways impact rotates the iliac wing inwards towards the opposite wing. This usually results in fracture of the sacrum or disruption of the sacro-iliac (SI) joints and simultaneous disruption of the pubic rami. These are often unstable fractures in a rotational plane but will normally maintain length in a vertical direction.

- Fractures of the sacrum. As well as lateral compression fractures, sacral fracture may result from falls from a height. Fractures may be displaced or undisplaced, and involvement of sacral nerve roots may occur with sensory and motor abnormalities (including saddle anaesthesia), and incontinence. Treatment is symptomatic with 2 or 3 weeks bed rest.

The neurological abnormalities are usually transient, but occasionally laminectomy may be required.

- Sacro-iliac joint disruption with fractures of the pubic rami. These fractures are associated with severe haemorrhage and damage to associated organs as well as to the diaphragm (due to raised intra-abdominal pressure). Treatment is directed towards stabilization of the pelvis using external or internal fixation.

2. *Fractures due to anterior forces.* Anterior forces result in 'open book' fractures (i.e. opening up of the pubic symphysis or fracture through the pubic rami. Disruption of the sacro-iliac joints may also occur, although these often remain intact as a hinge at the posterior aspect of the sacrum, allowing opening of the pelvis but again giving some degree of vertical stability. Fracture of all four pubic rami produces a 'floating segment' attached to the bladder and urethra. Urological problems are common. Treatment of open-book fractures is directed towards stabilization of the pelvis, usually by external fixation.

3. *Vertical shear forces.* These forces may result from a fall from a height and generally produce a vertical disruption of one hemi-pelvis relative to the other. Injuries of this kind are associated with severe soft-tissue trauma and marked instability when attempts at reduction are made. They may be associated with sacral fractures and neurological deficit. Treatment may include external fixation and, in selected cases, internal fixation with correction of vertical displacement.

Fractures of the acetabulum Fractures of the acetabulum are commonly associated with forces transmitted along the shaft of the femur and may therefore be associated with dislocation of the femoral head. They are also associated with lateral compression forces.

When the hip joint is markedly disrupted, open reduction with reconstruction and fixation of the fragments is the most appropriate treatment in order to restore congruity of the joint surface. However, if the acetabular floor is extremely comminuted, conservative treatment, with traction for approximately 6 weeks, may produce the best results.

Imaging

Plain radiographs of the pelvis taken during the primary survey will reveal most pelvic fractures. Discovery of a fracture of any part of the pelvic ring should immediately lead to a search for a reciprocal fracture in another part of the ring ('the polo mint' analogy suggests that it is impossible to crack a polo mint in one place only).

The radiograph should be studied in a logical manner, paying attention to the following:

- Is the film centred? Are the posterior spinous processes of the lumbar spine in the midline, and does a line pass along these and continue down the pubic symphysis?
- Is the outline of the sacrum clear and symmetrical? Is there any obvious distortion of the sacrum which might represent a fracture line?
- Are the sacro-iliac joints symmetrical? Do the SI joints look the same on both sides and is there any widening which can not be explained by malposition of the patient?
- Are the iliac crests symmetrical and at the same level?
- Are the obturator foramina symmetrical or do they look as if they have been rotated relative to one another?
- Is the acetabulum intact, or are there any signs of fracture? Is the hip dislocated or subluxed? Can the entire outline of the acetabulum be traced from posterior to anterior and are all parts of the acetabulum visible in order to exclude a fracture?

Further plain films may be required. Inlet or outlet views taken at 45° to the vertical (either looking down into the pelvis or up into the abdomen) exaggerate any antero-posterior displacement of pelvic fragments. Oblique views to assess the integrity of the anterior and posterior columns will be required in order to assess the acetabulum prior to reconstruction.

CT scanning is likely to be required before complex reconstructive pelvic surgery

Major fractures around the pubic rami may result in compound fractures that enter the urethra, bladder, vagina or rectum. These injuries require appropriate further imaging. If bladder perforation or urethral injury has occurred or is suspected, then either urethrography or cystography with water-soluble medium will be required.

Further reading

Dandy DJ. *Essential Orthopaedics and Trauma*, 2nd Edn. Edinburgh: Churchill Livingstone, 1993.

McRae R. *Practical Fracture Treatment*, 3rd Edn. Edinburgh: Churchill Livingstone, 1994.

Related topics of interest

PENETRATING CARDIAC INJURY

Penetrating cardiac injuries are particularly challenging as they require urgent invasive intervention if moribund patients are to be potentially salvageable; furthermore, in the multiply injured patient signs of such injuries may not be immediately apparent.

Incidence

The incidence of penetrating cardiac trauma varies according to the country, environment and method of injury. It is estimated that 3000 deaths per year occur due to gunshot wounds to the heart. The majority of penetrating cardiac wounds in the UK are due to stabbings.

Pathology

Blood loss depends on the chamber penetrated. Left ventricular penetration is more common than right and, due to the thicker muscle of the ventricular wall, small left ventricular penetrations may 'self-seal'.

Presentation

The classical presentation is of cardiac tamponade due to bleeding into the pericardial sac with compression of the heart. The following signs :

- Beck's triad (muffled heart sounds, elevated jugular venous pressure and hypotension),
- pulsus paradoxus (a decrease in systolic blood pressure of more than 10 mmHg during inspiration), and
- Kusmaul's sign [raised jugular venous pressure (JVP) on inspiration].

are rare (10–33% of cases), and are often difficult or impossible to elicit. In addition, hypovolaemia may mask elevation of the JVP. Other signs include:

- tachycardia, and
- electrical alternans on ECG.

Penetrating cardiac trauma may also present with devastating external haemorrhage or bleeding into the pleural cavity.

It is usually necessary, therefore, to assume that all patients with penetrating thoracic or upper abdominal injuries are at risk of penetrating cardiac trauma.

Investigations

The plain chest radiograph is usually normal in cardiac tamponade, due to the fibrous, non-distensible nature of the pericardial sac.

Subxiphoid pericardiocentesis is associated with a

significant rate of false negatives (25%) and is a potentially hazardous procedure. Some authorities contend that if cardiac arrest has occurred, immediate thoracotomy without pericardiocentesis is appropriate.

Transthoracic echocardiography is not completely reliable, and the investigation of choice is probably transoesophageal echocardiography; however, appropriateness of investigation of these patients must depend on:

- condition of the patient;
- skill and experience of the radiologist;
- availability of radiological facilities.

Treatment

1. Pre-operative. All patients should have minimal on-scene times, using a scoop and run policy. In particular, prolonged attempts at intravenous access should be delayed until the patient arrives in hospital. Intravenous fluids may worsen prognosis.

Time in the Accident and Emergency Department should be kept to a minimum and the unstable patient transferred to theatre as rapidly as possible. Pericardiocentesis should be regarded as a temporary measure, but was associated with a reduction in mortality from 94 to 63% if undertaken in A&E (25 to 17% if undertaken in theatre) (Callahan, 1984). The place of emergency-room thoracotomy is controversial, but evidence suggests that it is associated with occasional survivors in penetrating trauma, particularly if the patient still has vital signs on arriving in hospital. If thoracotomy is performed, bleeding can be controlled by digital pressure, insertion of a Foley catheter or horizontal mattress sutures, and cardiac compressions can be performed if necessary.

2. Operative.

- Wherever possible, surgery should be undertaken in theatre.
- For stable patients, median sternotomy is the incision of choice as it provides better access than antero-lateral thoracotomy. Wound extension is necessary in 2% of median sternotomies but 21% of antero-lateral thoracotomies.
- Cardiopulmonary bypass is only required in 2% of patients with penetrating cardiac trauma. It is usually needed for the repair of major proximal coronary artery injuries or where there is myocardial ischaemia. Repair

by direct suture or saphenous vein graft may be necessary.
- Coronary artery injuries are found in 3–9% of patients, the left anterior descending (LAD) artery being most commonly involved.

Prognosis

Penetrating cardiac injuries have a relatively better prognosis than blunt injuries of a similar severity. Factors associated with a good prognosis are:

- presence of vital signs;
- evidence of cardiac activity;
- patients with cardiac tamponade (prevents rapid loss of circulatory volume);
- stab wounds;
- isolated chest injuries;
- short pre-hospital times.

Factors associated with a poor prognosis are:

- no detectable vital signs;
- asystole;
- absent pupillary responses;
- associated extrathoracic injuries, especially head injuries.

Summary

The key features of the management of penetrating cardiac injuries are early clinical suspicion, rapid access to appropriate facilities and early surgery by skilled operators. Emergency-room thoracotomy may have a role to play in selected cases.

Further reading

Buckman P, *et al*. Penetrating cardiac wounds: prospective study of factors influencing initial resuscitation. *Journal of Trauma,* 1993; **34:** 717.

Callahan ML. Pericardiocentesis in traumatic and non-traumatic cardiac tamponade. *Annals of Emergency Medicine,* 1984; **17:** 924.

Jahangiri M, *et al*. Emergency thoracotomy for thoracic trauma in the accident and emergency department: indications and outcome. *Annals of the Royal College of Surgeons,* 1996; **78:** 221–2.

Related topics of interest

PERCUTANEOUS EMBOLIZATION IN PELVIC TRAUMA

Pelvic fractures are major contributing factors to death in patients with multiple injuries, estimates of mortality rates being between 9 and 19%. Bleeding and haematoma formation are frequent following pelvic ring disruption and result in shock and coagulopathy. Conventional external pelvic fixation may be inadequate to control severe bleeding. Percutaneous embolization is gaining increasing acceptance as a method of treating haemorrhage from pelvic trauma.

Investigation

Early embolization is clearly not appropriate in patients with obvious critical abdominal injuries or those who require exploratory laparotomy. Ultrasound or CT scanning may be used to exclude major solid viscus bleeding in the 'stable' patient. In pelvic fracture, small quantities of blood may seep through from an extraperitoneal haematoma and are responsible for the high false-positive rates in diagnostic peritoneal lavage (DPL).

Advantages of embolization

Angiographic examination and embolization avoids problems associated with open surgery:

- intraoperative loss of tamponade effect,
- massive intra-abdominal bleeding,
- surgical technical problems,
- inability to secure surgical haemostasis,

all of which contribute to the high mortality associated with this procedure in pelvic fractures.

Technique

- Angiography is usually performed via a catheter inserted into the femoral artery.
- Screening of the splenic, hepatic and mesenteric axes are routinely undertaken at the same time.
- Should the patient require an intravenous urogram, this must be performed after angiography in order not to compromise the vascular films.
- Embolization should be restricted to the bleeding artery only, thus ensuring collateral circulation. Occasionally a deteriorating patient may require a more radical life-saving embolization, (for example, of the internal iliac system).
- Embolization can be achieved with gel foam, poly-vinyl alcohol-calibrated particles and autologous clots. Different agents may be used in the same patient.

- Embolism should result in reversible embolization, reperfusion occurring as the patient recovers.

Gel foam and poly-vinyl alcohol have a half-life of a few weeks and are preferred to autologous clots which last only a few hours due to natural fibrinolysis.

Complications

There is a risk of urinary bladder or uterine necrosis after embolization of both hypogastric arteries: this risk must be weighed against the risks of ongoing haemorrhage. Patients with pelvic disruption may suffer perineal injuries and sacral plexus injury which may produce impotence. It is not yet known whether internal iliac embolization itself may produce impotence. Rhabdomyolysis has been reported.

Summary

Having excluded other causes of major haemorrhage, patients with severe or life-threatening bleeding from pelvic ring disruption may now be treated effectively by appropriate embolization.

Further reading

Piotin M, *et al.* Percutaneous transcatheter embolisation in pelvic ring disruption. *Injury,* 1995; **26** (10): 677–80.

Related topics of interest

PERIPHERAL NERVE INJURIES

Peripheral nerves, unlike nerves of the central nervous system, have the ability to regenerate after injury.

Anatomy

Peripheral nerves comprise three distinct anatomical components:

1. Fascicles. Bundles of myelinated and demyelinated nerve fibres held together by the connective tissue endoneurium.

2. Perineurium. A fibrous connective tissue sheath surrounding individual fascicles and imparting strength and resilience to them.

3. Epineurium. A connective tissue matrix binding fascicles together and condensing externally to form the epineural sheath.

The blood supply to peripheral nerves is from the surrounding tissue along the course of the nerve.

Regeneration

Following division of a peripheral nerve the axon and myelin sheath degenerate in a retrograde fashion for several centimetres (Wallerian degeneration). Several days after the injury, new axons begin to grow out from the proximal end and grow distally; the rate of growth being 1–3 mm/day. If the connective tissue framework of the nerve is intact and in continuity then nerve regeneration may occur. In a mixed nerve the correct reconnection of sensory and motor nerves to their end organs is an entirely random process.

Mechanism of nerve injury

- Compression (e.g. of the common peroneal nerve by an incorrectly applied below-knee plaster).
- Traction (e.g. of the brachial plexus in motor cycle injuries).
- Ischaemia (e.g. of forearm nerves after prolonged application of a surgical tourniquet).
- Laceration (e.g. the median at the wrist following penetrating glass injuries).

The management of peripheral nerve injuries is influenced by the extent of injury. Injuries may be classified into three broad groups (after Seddon's classification):

1. Neurapraxia. This is contusion of the nerve caused by direct blunt trauma. It is characterized by:

- Conduction block.
- An intact axon.
- Absence of Wallerian degeneration.
- Spontaneous recovery.

2. Axonotmesis. This is characterized by a crush injury or stretching injury leading to:

- Degeneration of the axon.
- Intact connective tissue nerve sheath.
- Spontaneous recovery.

Because the injury is more severe than in neurapraxia, recovery is less predictable and when present may be incomplete.

3. Neuronotmesis. This is characterized by a penetrating or incised wound leading to:

- Division of the nerve (partial or complete).
- Degeneration of the nerve distal to the lesion.
- No recovery.

Recovery in such injuries does not occur without surgical intervention.

In the case of neurapraxia, axonotmesis and neuronotmesis after surgical repair, recovery may be delayed for several months. Active physiotherapy to maintain normal joint movement and muscle, tendon and ligament length is required if maximal recovery is to be expected.

Diagnosis

Diagnosis of peripheral nerve injury depends upon taking an adequate history to determine the mechanism of injury. This will suggest the probability that the lesion is a neuronotmesis, which requires active surgical intervention, or a neurapraxia or axonotmesis which can be managed conservatively.

Clinical examination

Clinical examination should be directed to establishing any deficit in:

1. Motor function. The motor supply of all nerves traversing the injury site and supplying muscles distal to the injury should be examined.

2. *Sensation.* Any deficit in the sensory supply to the skin distal to the injury should be sought. Complete loss of sensation may not be present soon after an injury. Sensation should be compared with the contralateral side to establish any qualitative difference. Any such difference should be taken to indicate a nerve lesion.

3. *Sweating.* Interruption of the nerve supply to the skin causes an immediate loss of sweating in the area of supply of that nerve. This is frequently the earliest sign of a nerve lesion. The easiest way to detect such loss of sweating is to draw a plastic pen across the skin. In normal skin there is some resistance to the movement. In the presence of a nerve lesion the resistance is lost.

4. *Two point blunt discrimination.* In the pulp skin of the fingers the normal range of separation for discrimination is 3–5 mm. Any increase in this distance is abnormal. This test is particularly useful in partial nerve lesions.

In the case of a penetrating or incised wound any nerve in the vicinity of such injuries should be assumed to be damaged until proven otherwise. In young children and others who are difficult to assess formal exploration may be needed to exclude a nerve lesion.

Management

In all cases where neuronotmesis is suspected formal exploration should be undertaken. The repair should, where possible, be undertaken early as a primary procedure.

1. *Contraindications to primary repair.*

- The presence of other injuries requiring more immediate management.
- Patient unfit for operation.
- Presence of infection.
- Nerve injury due to missile injuries.
- Non-availability of a surgeon experienced in nerve repair. It is generally agreed that nerve repair should be undertaken by a surgeon experienced in the use of an operating microscope using either the epineural repair or group fascicular repair techniques.

2. *Factors influencing outcome from nerve repair.*

- Accuracy of axial alignment of the nerve.

- Fascicular apposition.
- Degree of suture line fibrosis.

Further reading

Burge P. Peripheral nerve injuries. *Surgery*, 1990; 2059–63.

Related topics of interest

PNEUMATIC ANTI-SHOCK GARMENT (PASG/MAST SUIT)

The earliest description of a pneumatic anti-shock garment is from 1903, however these garments did not come into widespread clinical use until after their rediscovery during World War II when garments of this kind were used as antigravity suits (G suits) to prevent loss of consciousness in fighter pilots. Currently pneumatic anti-shock garments are more widely used in the USA and South Africa than they are in the UK.

Physiological mechanisms of action

The physiological actions of the PASG are controversial, no current consensus of opinion exists but the following have been suggested:

- Autotransfusion of blood from the legs: estimates of the volume transfused vary from 200 ml to 25% of the available blood volume.
- Increase in peripheral vascular resistance.
- Mobilization of blood pooled in the lower extremities, abdomen or engorged muscles.
- Redistribution of cardiac output because of reduced blood flow to the legs and abdomen.
- Tamponade of bleeding vessels.
- Splintage of fractures.

Other physiological effects of the PASG include increased venous return, decreased vital capacity, increased pulmonary wedge pressure, decreased renal perfusion and metabolic acidosis. In normal (e.g. non-shocked) people application of a PASG results in a rise in blood pressure, stroke volume and cardiac output.

Indications

1. *Shock.*

- Hypovolaemic (especially due to pelvic or lower limb fractures). It has been suggested that the PASG should only be used in hypovolaemic shock if the BP is less than 90 mmHg.
- Neurogenic.
- Anaphylactic.
- Septic.

2. *Splintage of pelvic and lower limb fractures.*

3. *Crush injuries.* The PASG can be used as a 'portable compression' to prevent or reduce the effects of metabolic toxins following release.

The PASG will also be effective in reducing the hypotensive effects of sudden removal of weight from the legs or lower body.

Contraindications

1. Absolute (controversial).

- Left ventricular failure.
- Pulmonary oedema.

2. Relative.

- Ruptured diaphragm (suspected or confirmed). Consider inflating the leg compartments only.
- Congestive cardiac failure.
- Cardiac injury.
- Thoracic vascular injury.
- CNS injury/head injury.

Use of the PASG

The PASG is normally laid out flat on a scoop stretcher and the patient placed on it after extrication. Each leg compartment is inflated individually, followed, if necessary, by inflation of the abdominal compartment. Compartments are usually inflated to about 30–50 mmHg with further increases based on monitoring the blood pressure. If the suit is inflated to maximum pressure (i.e. after the safety valves have operated) this pressure should only be maintained for about 30 min.

Inflation

Inflation of the leg compartments should only be considered in the following circumstances:

- Pregnancy (more than 26 weeks gestation).
- Abdominal evisceration or impalement.
- Suspected or actual diaphragmatic rupture.

The legs of the PASG may be shortened by rolling back before use.

Deflation

Most of the problems which have prevented widespread use of the PASG in the UK occur on deflation. The majority of A&E staff in the UK (nursing and medical) are not familiar with the PASG and therefore unless specific expertise is available, the responsibility for removing the garment remains with the doctor who applied it. The PASG should not be removed until:

- Two large IV lines are *in situ* with transfusion/infusion in progress.
- Monitoring of vital signs is available.
- The patient is in the operating theatre.
- The patient is haemodynamically stable.

The compartments of the PASG are slowly deflated, one at a time, beginning with the abdominal compartment. If the blood pressure falls by more than 5 mmHg deflation is stopped and the blood pressure restored by infusion before deflation is recommenced. Attempts have been made in A&E to cut PASGs off, not only is this expensive but the cardiovascular consequences may be catastrophic. Similar problems may result from accidental puncture of the suit on a sharp object at the scene of an accident.

X-rays, catheterization, rectal and vaginal examinations are all possible with a PASG in place.

One effect of transferring a patient by air in a PASG is to increase the pressure from a mast suit as the altitude rises (due to air expansion within the suit) and perhaps more importantly to lower it as the altitude falls. This is not usually a problem with low altitude helicopter transfer.

Complications

- Compartment syndrome.
- Stimulation of:
  (a) Micturition.
  (b) Defaecation.
  (c) Vomiting.
- Increased bleeding from areas not covered by suit (e.g. the thorax).
- Respiratory embarrassment and dyspnoea (abdominal compartment).
- Limited access to abdomen.

Conclusion

'The jury remains out' on PASGs, but even within the UK there are passionate advocates of their use. It seems likely that they do (albeit rarely) have a role in the management of hypovolaemia due to pelvic and lower limb fractures. A similar effect can, of course, result from the patient's own motor cycle leathers or even tight jeans which should only be removed if there is a compelling reason to do so.

Further reading

Clancy MJ. Pneumatic anti-shock garment — does it have a future? *Journal of Accident and Emergency Medicine*, 1995; **12**(2): 123–5.

Related topics of interest

PREGNANCY AND TRAUMA

Trauma in pregnancy presents a unique and challenging task to the trauma team. The priorities for treatment remain the same as for the non-pregnant patient, the outcome for the foetus being dependent in the majority of cases upon the survival of the mother. An obstetrician and experienced anaesthetist should be involved early to maximize the chance of survival for both mother and foetus.

A number of anatomical and physiological changes occur in pregnancy which serve to modify the approach to the pregnant trauma victim.

Anatomical changes

The uterus is an intra-pelvic organ in the first 12 weeks of pregnancy and is therefore protected from direct injury by the bony pelvis. By the 24th week of pregnancy the uterus has risen to the level of the umbilicus and by the 36th week to the level of the costal margin. Thereafter as the head engages the uterus descends. During foetal growth the intestines are displaced to the upper part of the abdominal cavity.

In early pregnancy the muscular uterus is thick walled, and the relatively small foetus is protected by a large volume of amniotic fluid. As pregnancy proceeds and the foetus grows, the uterine wall becomes thinner and the relative volume of amniotic fluid falls thus reducing the cushioning effect to the foetus.

The placenta is a relatively inelastic structure, so shearing forces to the abdomen such as those occurring in blunt trauma, in particular seat belt injuries, can lead to abruptio placentae.

Physiological changes

These will be considered under the headings of the systems they affect.

1. Airway. Passive regurgitation and aspiration risk is increased by:

- Delayed gastric emptying.
- Relaxation of the gastro-oesophageal sphincter.

Early placement of a nasogastric tube, and consideration of early endotracheal intubation with application of cricoid pressure are indicated. Endotracheal intubation is more difficult due to:

- Subglottic oedema.
- Breast enlargement.

2. *Breathing.* Hypoxia is more likely because of increased oxygen consumption. Pre-oxygenation and monitoring with a pulse oximeter are required during intubation. Ventilation is more difficult due to:

- Increased chest compliance.
- Splinting of the diaphragm by the uterus.

The physiological hyperventilation of pregnancy caused by increased tidal volume, leads to a respiratory alkalosis:

- $paCO_2$ falls to 4 kPa.
- $paCO_2$ of 5.3 kPa indicates maternal and therefore foetal acidosis.

3. *Circulation.* The following circulatory changes occur:

- Cardiac output increased by 1.5–2.0 l/min.
- Blood volume increased by 40–50%.
- Resting heart rate increased by 15–20 b/min.
- Systolic and diastolic BP decreased by 5–15 mmHg.
- Haematocrit falls to 31–35%.

The normal physiological response to hypovolaemic shock will be attenuated, up to 30–35% of circulating volume may be lost before clinical signs of shock appear (tachycardia, hypotension and increased respiratory rate). Hypovolaemic shock in the pregnant woman leads to a preferential reduction in uteroplacental blood to the benefit of the mother and detriment of the foetus.

Compression of the inferior vena cava by the pregnant uterus (aortocaval compression) may lead to a reduction in venous return by as much as 30–40%. This can be prevented by:

- Tilting the patient left side down.
- Manually displacing the uterus to the left.

Primary survey

1. *Airway.* Airway control with immobilization of the cervical spine is carried out as for the non-pregnant patient and supplemental oxygen is administered. If spinal injury has been excluded the patient is managed on her left-hand side by inserting a wedge under the right hip. If spinal injury has not been excluded manual displacement of the uterus to the left can be performed.

2. *Breathing.* If the patient is not breathing and protective airway reflexes are impaired then endotracheal intubation

with application of cricoid pressure should be considered. Increased ventilatory pressures may be required to overcome increased chest compliance and diaphragmatic splinting.

3. Circulation. Early volume replacement is indicated even if the mother appears physiologically stable. This is because increased maternal plasma volume delays the onset of clinical signs of shock, therefore the foetus may be shocked even if the mother appears stable.

Secondary survey

This proceeds as for the non-pregnant patient. In addition assessment of the uterus and foetus is required including assessment of foetal movements and doppler assessment of foetal heart sounds. In later pregnancy cardiotochography can be used. Ultrasound examination of the foetus, placenta and amniotic fluid provides additional information on viability and the presence of, and the degree of trauma to the foetus and uterus.

Relevant X-ray examination should not be withheld because of fear of exposure of the foetus. Where possible abdominal shielding will reduce the dose of X-rays to the foetus.

Blood should be taken for the Kleinhauer test to assess the presence and degree of foetomaternal haemorrhage. The presence of foetomaternal haemorrhage in a rhesus negative mother is an indication for prophylactic Anti-D.

All pregnant women suffering trauma, no matter how apparently trivial the degree, warrant obstetric or gynaecological assessment. Placental abruption may occur up to 48 hours after the injury and present with few signs initially.

Beyond 26 weeks a foetus is potentially viable, therefore even if the mother is not responding to resuscitation or is apparently dead, resuscitation should be continued until obstetric assessment is carried out. Emergency caesarian section in this situation may result in the delivery of a viable foetus.

Further reading

American College of Surgeons Committee on Trauma. Abdominal Trauma. In: *Advanced Trauma Life Support: Program for Physicians*. Chicago: American College of Surgeons, 1993; 141–58.

Robertson C, Redmond AD. *The Management of Major Trauma.* Oxford Handbooks in Emergency Medicine. Oxford: Oxford University Press, 1991.

Skinner D, Driscoll P, Earlam R. *ABC of Major Trauma.* London: BMJ Publications, 1991; 46–50.

Related topics of interest

Abdominal injuries (p. 1)
Pelvic fractures (p. 224)
Pneumatic anti-shock garment (PASG/MAST suit) (p. 238)

PREVENTABLE DEATHS

Of all deaths in the UK, 2.5% are due to trauma. Trauma is the most common cause of death in the UK in patients aged between 1 and 45 years, and the cause of 61% of all deaths between the ages of 15 and 24. Yet a Royal College of Surgeons Report in 1988 suggested that 33% of all trauma deaths were preventable.

Potential causes of preventable deaths

A recent study (Gorman *et al.*, 1996) identified the following problems in head-injured patients who suffered preventable deaths:

- operative delay, 35%;
- no operation for mass lesion, 65%.

and in non-head-injured patients who suffered preventable deaths:

- missed injuries, 67%;
- poor airway care, 57%;
- delayed or no operation, 52%;
- undertransfusion, 38%;
- inadequate surgery, 19%.

Statistics

1.   Head injury. Recent studies suggest that between 13% and 47% of deaths due to head injury are preventable. A mistaken diagnosis of alcoholic intoxication or cerebrovascular accident rather than intracranial haematoma is estimated to be responsible for between 39% and 66% of these preventable deaths. Other contributing factors are believed to be delayed or absent neurosurgical intervention and inadequate care of the airway.

2.   Blunt trauma in general. A number of recent British studies suggest that the preventable death rate in blunt trauma is approximately 16% (22% if head injury deaths are excluded). If this figure is correct, then it suggests that 638 potentially preventable blunt trauma deaths occur each year in England and Wales, or 38 deaths in each regional health authority.

3.   Penetrating trauma. The estimated numbers of preventable deaths due to penetrating trauma in the UK are, not surprisingly, much lower than for blunt trauma. An estimate of 19 such deaths per year has been made.

4. *Preventable deaths during pre-hospital care.* It has been suggested in a recent study from America that 12% of patients suffered preventable deaths due to errors in their pre-hospital management. In particular, problems were identified with unnecessary delays for intravenous access, intubation and the application of pneumatic anti-shock garments (PASG/MAST suit).

5. *Preventable deaths in children.* A recent study of trauma deaths in children (Wyatt *et al.*, 1997) suggests that the majority of children dying from trauma are either dead when found or die at the scene of the accident before receiving medical intervention. This must have implications for initiatives designed to reduce death rates from trauma amongst children, which need to emphasize education and accident prevention.

Solutions

There is some evidence from American figures to suggest that the introduction of specialist trauma centres can effect a significant reduction in preventable deaths from trauma. However, there are differences in the epidemiology of American trauma and the structure of trauma care in the USA (other than the presence of trauma centres) which mean that this data is not directly comparable to the UK. Estimates of the fall in preventable deaths following the introduction of specialist trauma centres vary from 19% (a fall from 34% to 15%) to 50% (a fall from 71% to 21%).

It is likely that attempts to diminish delays in time to definitive care, as well as attention to simple resuscitation priorities, will reduce the incidence of preventable deaths. In particular, on-scene times should be kept to a minimum, inappropriate interventions and misdiagnoses avoided, and rapid access to definitive surgical care expedited.

A key priority in the reduction of preventable deaths from trauma must be the implementation of patient education and accident prevention initiatives, especially in reducing deaths from road-traffic accidents.

Further reading

Anderson ID, *et al.* Retrospective study of 1000 deaths from injury in England and Wales. *British Medical Journal,* 1988; **296:** 1305.
Gorman DF, *et al.* Preventable deaths among major trauma patients in Mersey region, North Wales and the Isle of Man. *Injury,* 1996; **27:** 189–92.

Jennett B, Carlin J. Preventable mortality and morbidity after head injury. *Injury,* 1978; **10:** 31.

Wyatt JP, *et al.* Timing of paediatric deaths after trauma. *British Medical Journal,* 1997; **314:** 868.

Related topics of interest

PSYCHOLOGICAL ASPECTS OF TRAUMA

Historical records, particularly of military combat, confirm that trauma damages psychologically as well as physically. Too often, however, victims are ostracized, criticized and ignored. Even survivors of the Nazi concentration camps were met with a 'conspiracy of silence', and, most significantly, even their medical records often made no mention of their experiences during the Holocaust.

Ignorance, malice and, perhaps, even jealousy may sometimes account for this denial of the suffering of others, but a more likely reason is the need to maintain certain assumptions about ourselves and our world. We like to believe in our own capacity to face with dignity the vicissitudes of life in an orderly, predictable world in which we are the architects of our own destiny. Catastrophic events and the suffering of others challenge these cherished assumptions because they suggest that we too might be in the position of a hapless victim. Sadly, by blaming victims or dismissing their suffering because they are 'wimps' or are seeking sympathy and compensation we inflict upon them a 'second injury'.

Post-traumatic stress disorder (PTSD)

A landmark was reached in 1980 when this term was introduced by the American Psychiatric Association into the third edition of the *Diagnostic and Statistical Manual* (DSM-III). This step:

- introduced some order into the taxonomy of trauma-related conditions;
- legitimized the suffering of victims not only of military and major civilian catastrophes but of the personal trauma of daily life (e.g. road-traffic accidents (RTAs) and assaults);
- sired much needed research into the aetiology, phenomenology and treatment of post-traumatic syndromes.

In 1992 the concept also appeared in the tenth revision of the *International Classification of Disease* (ICD-10), in conjunction with several other stress-related disorders.

(a) Acute stress reaction. This is a transient disorder which usually subsides within hours or days. No one type of symptom dominates; it involves a fluctuating picture of depression, anxiety, anger, despair, withdrawal, numbness and overactivity.

(b) Post-traumatic stress disorder. This may be an acute, chronic or delayed reaction to a 'stressful event or situation... of an exceptionally threatening or catastrophic nature, which is likely to cause pervasive distress in almost anyone...'. The characteristic symptoms are intrusive in nature, e.g. flashback and nightmares, against a sense of numbness and emotional blunting, detachment from others, unresponsiveness and avoidance. 'Commonly' there is fear and avoidance of reminders of the trauma, and 'often' there is hyperarousal with hypervigilance, an exaggerated startle response and insomnia. These symptoms must have endured for at least 1 month, and the diagnosis is not usually made unless it can be demonstrated that it arose within 6 months of the event.

(c) Adjustment disorders. These entail distress and emotional disturbance of a severity which interferes with normal adjustment. There are different subcategories reflecting the primary disturbance. Generally, the onset is within 1 month of the trauma, and they do not usually endure for more than 6 months (with the exception of 'prolonged depressive reaction' which can endure up to 2 years). Subcategories:

- Brief depressive reaction.
- Prolonged depressive reaction.
- Mixed anxiety and depressive reaction.
- With predominant disturbance of other emotions.
- With predominant disturbance of conduct.
- With predominant disturbance of emotion and conduct.

(d) Dissociative disorders. These include dissociative amnesia, dissociative fugue and dissociative disorders of movement and sensation (previously called 'hysterical conversion disorder'). The common denominator among these conditions is a partial or complete loss of the normal integration between memories of the past, awareness of one's identity and sensations and bodily control. They occur unconsciously in response to overwhelming stressful or traumatic experiences (or sometimes chronic intolerable life circumstances). The onset in response to trauma is usually sudden, and they tend to remit after weeks and months following that event or situation.

(e) Enduring personality change after a catastrophic experience. Certain trauma, either by virtue of their severity or prolongation, may induce a permanent change in personality, characterized by a hostile and suspicious attitude to the world, social withdrawal, feelings of emptiness or hopelessness and a chronic sense of 'being on edge' (major disasters, being taken hostage, being tortured and incarceration in concentration camps are experiences which might have such an effect).

Prevalence of PTSD

Community surveys suggest a lifetime risk of 1% (about the same as that for schizophrenia). Estimates for specific trauma are as follows: rape (35%); 'battered women' (45%); burn injuries (45%); RTA victims (10%); major flood (28%, even after 14 years); terrorist attacks (18%); Falkland War Veterans (22%) and major transportation disasters (50%).

Prognostic indicators

No single trauma is a necessary and sufficient condition for a post-traumatic syndrome. The following increase the risk and relate to poor outcome after traumatic events.

- Prolonged exposure to the trauma (e.g. being trapped or being taken hostage or because of serial exposure to different trauma).
- (Perceived) threat to life (i.e. the threat may be in the eye of the beholder).
- Multiple deaths and/or mutilation.
- Sudden and unexpected events (because there is no time to prepare).
- Special meaning (e.g. children victims or identification with the victims and their families).
- Concurrent life stresses. (Perhaps before discharging patients from trauma units we should ask not just 'Have you somebody to go home to?' but also 'What are you going home to?')
- Previous experience of trauma. (This can, however, have a complex relationship to adjustment. It can have an 'immunizing' effect, particularly if the victims believed they coped well previously, but it can also have a cumulative or sensitizing effect. Rape, for instance, usually leaves the victim more vulnerable to psychiatric illness in the event of a subsequent sexual assault.)
- Severity of personal injury. (This factor may be more related to the personal significance of the injury rather than to how it is defined objectively.)
- Lack of social, professional and family support.
- Extreme early reactions to trauma. (Those who display features of an 'acute stress reaction' are more likely to develop PTSD.)

- Miscellaneous. (Early parental loss, low educational level, personality traits, female gender, younger age and previous personal and family history of psychiatric illness commonly (but not universally) correlate with poor post-traumatic adjustment.)

Duration of PTSD

Without treatment it may endure for years, and physically injured patients may worsen after discharge. Certain neurobiological and psychological changes may be permanent such that vulnerability to subsequent mental illness (including further episodes of PTSD) is increased. The most malignant and chronic form of PTSD may result in marked social decline. It is one of the most common conditions found among the homeless. Litigation and compensation have little bearing on the presentation of symptoms or on their chronicity.

Co-morbidity

PTSD is frequently accompanied by other disorders, particularly depression, generalized anxiety, phobia and substance abuse. Also, PTSD patients are more likely than non-sufferers to have additional medical problems such as hypertension.

Treatment of post-traumatic syndromes

Proposed treatments are legion; randomized control trials are a rarity. Many new treatments are simply old wine in new bottles (and not even of vintage stock). Reported outcomes vary (possibly due in part to the complex level of co-morbidity associated with PTSD), but the following are guidelines:

1. Pharmacotherapy. No single compound or class of drug addresses the full spectrum of post-traumatic symptoms but:

- Tricyclic antidepressants and monoamine oxidase inhibitors alleviate intrusive phenomena but have little effect on avoidant symptoms.
- The new SSRIs (e.g. fluoxetine) may help avoidant symptoms but drug-induced insomnia may be a problem (PTSD patients are particularly sensitive to side-effects).
- Benzodiazepines may play a useful role in the early stages (e.g. to deal with an acute stress reaction) but have little effect on the core PTSD symptoms.
- The anticonvulsants carbamazepine and valproate may help with insomnia and the re-experiencing phenomena

and with hyperarousal and avoidant/numbing symptoms, respectively.

- Autonomic hyper-reactivity may respond to clonidine and propranolol.
- Neuroleptics have no role as frontline treatments except in the cases of psychotic behaviour and overwhelming aggressive and/or self-destructive behaviour.

2. *Psychotherapy.* Many of the reported successes (largely from open trials and anecdotal evidence) associated with a range of such interventions are probably much due to the impact of 'non-specific factors' rather than to any ingredient specific to a particular therapy. The most persuasive evidence is in favour of those treatments which involve:

- exposure to the original stressor or reminders thereof (e.g. flooding, graded exposure), and
- helping patients to alter the meaning of the trauma and its sequelae (e.g. cognitive behavioural therapy).

Clinical experience also suggests that group therapy (including self-help groups) is of value by providing mutual support, 'education', shared problem-solving, reassurance, and social and political action. Such groups may be valuable also for families and spouses.

More recently, enthusiastic claims have been made for eye movement desensitization and reprocessing therapy, but its theoretical basis has yet to be formulated convincingly, and randomized control trials are required.

Normal reactions to trauma 'Normal' and 'pathological' reactions lie on a continuum. They are generally distinguished by the extent to which they render patients dysfunctional in terms of their adjustment to the demands of normal life. The following are commonly observed in trauma victims, particularly in the short term.

1. *Numbness and denial.* A natural protection against being overwhelmed. However, this may also prevent patients taking in what staff tell them.

2. *Fear.* Essential to the initiation of the 'fight/flight' response. Patients should be reassured that there is no need to feel ashamed of being afraid.

3. *Depression.* Commonly seen in relation to loss.

4. *Elation.* Similar to 'combat rush' described by war veterans. This is probably due to a combination of psychological factors (e.g. at having survived) and neuroendocrinological ones. (This may lead temporarily to a raised pain threshold.)

5. *Anger.* This may be redirected on to those who carry out painful treatment procedures or who have to break bad news to trauma victims.

6. *Helplessness.* A sense of powerlessness and helplessness is pathognomic of the traumatized victim. If prolonged it can lead to excessive dependency.

7. *Guilt.* 'Survivor' guilt is common after multiple fatalities when survivors believe (usually wrongly) that they were responsible for the deaths of others. Parents too often experience this in relation to the death of a child (e.g. in an RTA). This guilt may explain the increased risks of violent death by homicide, suicide and RTAs reported in combat veterans.

8. *Irritability.* A pernicious problem at home and at work, that can strain otherwise loving and caring relationships. It is probably due to a combination of anger, frustration (at the trauma) and autonomic hypersensitivity.

9. *Cognitive changes.* Victims commonly misperceive the order in which, and the speed at which, events occur during trauma. (Most commonly they see everything as having been slowed down.) In addition, they frequently display 'tunnel vision' such that even important events and circumstances occurring peripherally may not be registered.

10. *Impaired sleep.* This is associated with autonomic hyperarousal and hypervigilance. Sleep is commonly punctuated by nightmares which may deter patients from trying to sleep. The sleep architecture is altered: increased proportion of light sleep (stages 1 and 2); decreased deep sleep ('delta' sleep) and increased REM sleep.

11. Flashbacks. These are involuntary re-experiencing of the original trauma and its associated emotions. They may involve any or all sensory modalities.

12. Autonomic hyperarousal (and hypervigilance). These may have biological survival value but they can be distressing to patients causing them to over-react to sensory input. (Alcohol is commonly used as a form of self-medication for this symptom.)

13. Avoidant behaviour. Patients seek to avoid all reminders of the trauma by not talking about it, by not reading about it or by avoiding situations or people reminiscent of the trauma. (Because this can become a major problem in the longer term, collusion by staff with patients' total avoidance is not desirable.)

NB: The last three reactions (flashbacks, hyperarousal and avoidance) are the distinguishing features of PTSD according to both DSM-IV and ICD-10, but only if they have endured for at least 1 month.

Guidelines

There are guidelines to identify patients who may be having difficulty in coping (despite what they themselves say).

1. Excessive denial and numbness. This is a problem when it causes patients to refuse to adhere to the treatment regimen.

2. Repeated carelessness and minor accidents. Concentration and short-term recall commonly suffer a decline after trauma and can contribute to such effects.

3. Changes in work performance. Some victims display a decrement in work performance; others submerge themselves in their work to an obsessive extent.

4. Overindulgences. Apart from working to excess, trauma patients may over indulge in food, tobacco, alcohol and other psychoactive substances.

5. *Russian roulette*. Despite having survived a life-threatening event some victims, at work or while driving their cars or during leisure, can be seen to be taking risks.

Trauma staff, emergency personnel and other 'helpers'

Substantial evidence now exists to indicate that 'helpers' can become secondary victims who may display any of the reactions, symptoms and syndromes described above. In addition, they may show:

- An inability to 'let go' of the trauma (causing them to talk endlessly about it or even to seek out further similar incidents in which to become involved).
- An inability to 'let go' of relationships. (Adversity can bond people together. Such relationships may, however, threaten family and marital ones.)
- 'Compassion fatigue' (helping trauma victims is rewarding but it can also be draining).

Debriefing

Because of the potentially disabling effects of dealing with traumatic events and their victims, there has been a move towards providing 'debriefing' after what are generically called 'critical incidents'. There are different models of debriefing, but their general aims are to:

- normalize individuals' reactions;
- enable the cathartic expression of emotions;
- reinforce the strength of the group;
- identify positive gains from the incident;
- help individuals to disengage from the incident.

The following principles should also be recognized; debriefing:

- is not psychotherapy;
- should be used only by trained personnel;
- is a group process;
- should be used approximately 24–72 hours after the incident;
- is a preventative procedure for normal individuals after an abnormal event.

Generally, participants in professionally conducted debriefing sessions report favourably upon their experiences therein. Evaluative research is, however, urgently required to demonstrate that such a procedure is psychoprophylactic and prevents the subsequent emergence of psychopathology.

Conclusion
- Traumatic events are unquestionably a source of psychopathology and extensive suffering for victims and their families. Vulnerability to adverse reactions and to problems of adjustment is a function of certain features of the trauma and of the victims' background, personality and current circumstances.
- 'At-risk' guidelines should be used to involve the early intervention of mental health professionals.
- Effective treatment for post-traumatic syndromes are available, but much more evaluation of such interventions is required to establish their therapeutic and prophylactic value.

Further reading

Alexander DA. Trauma research: a new era (editorial). *Journal of Psychosomatic Research,* 1996; **41** (1): 1–5.

Gibson M. *Order From Chaos.* Birmingham: Venture Press, 1991.

Mayou RA, Duthie R. Psychiatric consequences of road traffic accidents. *British Medical Journal,* 1993; **307:** 647–51.

Mitchell JT, Everly GS. *Critical Incident Stress Debriefing: CISD.* Ellicot City: Chevron Publishing, 1995.

Wilson JP, Raphael B. *International Handbook of Traumatic Stress Syndromes.* New York: Plenum Press, 1993.

Related topics of interest

PULSE OXIMETRY

The pulse oximeter uses the technique of spectrophotometry to give a continuous non-invasive measure of arterial oxygen saturation and pulse rate. This allows continuous monitoring for the presence of hypoxaemia in situations where intermittent estimation of invasively derived arterial blood gases is either impossible or undesirable.

Function of the pulse oximeter The pulse oximeter relies upon the differential absorption of red and infrared light by oxyhaemoglobin and deoxyhaemoglobin (usually 660 nm (red), the wavelength at which the absorption difference between the two molecules is greatest, and 940 nm (infrared), the control wavelength) to derive a value for saturation from an empirically derived nomogram within its processor unit. The accuracy of the pulse oximeter when compared to directly measured saturation is ± 2–3%.

Operation A probe is placed across a digit, ear lobe or across the nasal bridge. The probe consists of two light-emitting diodes (one red and one infrared emitting) and a detector. The two light sources shine light across the interposed tissue to be absorbed by the detector. A proportion of each wavelength is absorbed; the differential absorption depending upon the relative proportions of each type of haemoglobin present. The processor separates the light component absorbed by the tissues in the steady state from that absorbed at maximal pulsation of the tissue. The assumption is made that that extra absorption occuring at maximal pulsation is due to absorption by the arterial component of the blood. Calculated saturation at this point gives a measure of arterial rather than mixed arterial and venous saturation.

Uses of pulse oximetry Early detection of hypoxaemia: studies have shown that the correlation between cyanosis and hypoxaemia is poor, patients may not appear cyanosed until saturations have fallen well below 90%.

Indication of poor peripheral perfusion (e.g. shock, arterial occlusion, compartment syndrome, hypothermia): because the processor separates out the pulsatile component of the blood flow, poor peripheral perfusion will result in a failure to read a saturation level, with consequent triggering of the alarm.

Measurement of systolic blood pressure in low flow states: a cuff is gradually inflated proximal to the oximeter probe placed on a digit, the point at which the signal fails to be detected correlates well with the systolic blood pressure.

Allen's test: the presence of a signal with application of the probe to the index finger and occlusion of the radial artery indicates the presence of an intact palmar arterial arch.

Differentiation of true tonic–clonic seizures from pseudoseizures: in pseudoseizures the saturation will remain normal, in tonic–clonic seizures it will fall.

Disadvantages of the pulse oximeter

- Often fails to function when the patient is shocked, limiting its usefulness in acute trauma (although this may be seen as advantageous in indicating poor perfusion).

- It is unreliable in the presence of dyshaemoglobins (e.g. carboxyhaemoglobin, methaemoglobin). This is of particular importance in victims of carbon monoxide poisoning where a false sense of security can be engendered in the presence of an apparently normal saturation. In any situation in which carbon monoxide poisoning is suspected, the paO_2 should be measured using a blood gas analyser and the carboxyhaemoglobin level measured using a CO-oximeter. In the presence of methaemoglobinaemia and the absence of hypoxia, the oximetric saturation tends towards 85%.

- Gives no indication of ventilatory adequacy: in patients receiving supplementary oxygen the saturation may be normal in the presence of significant hypercarbia, in any situation where ventilatory failure is suspected, or the hypoxic patient fails to respond to adequate oxygenation, arterial blood gases should be measured.

- There is a non-linear relationship between SpO_2 and paO_2: under normal conditions an SpO_2 of 94–95% correlates with a paO_2 of 10 kPa; between 95% and 100% saturation large changes in paO_2 correlate with small changes in SpO_2, below this level relatively small changes in paO_2 correlate with large changes in SpO_2. The correlation between SpO_2 and paO_2 varies with a left or right shift of the oxygen dissociation curve.

- Delay in detecting falls in saturation: machines from different manufacturers use different sampling methods when displaying saturation levels, this can

lead to appreciable delays in detecting falls in saturation.
- Functions poorly in the presence of movement: this may be partly overcome by using machines which also detect changes in the ECG to compensate for extraneous motion.
- Extrinsic light may interfere with the accuracy of the sensor, leading to over-reading of saturation: this is overcome by shielding the probe from extraneous light sources.
- Some types of nail varnish (usually metallic) will interfere with the transmission of light across the probe.
- Severe anaemia: there may be insufficient haemoglobin present for the sensor to function.

Further reading

Moyle JTB. *Pulse Oximetry*. Principles and Practice Series. London: BMJ Publishing Group, 1994.

Related topics of interest

Anaesthesia (p. 21)
Invasive monitoring (p. 170)
Laparoscopy and thoracoscopy in trauma (p. 181)
Shock (p. 261)
Thoracic trauma (p. 295)

SHOCK

Shock may be defined as a condition in which the circulating fluid volume is insufficient to meet the metabolic needs of the tissues.

The management priorities for the shocked patient follow the same priorities as for all trauma namely ABC. Although shock may not be formally identified or classified until circulatory assessment has been performed, respiratory causes of shock (tension pneumothorax and flail chest) may be identified and treated when breathing is assessed.

Classification of shock

1. Hypovolaemic. An absolute reduction in circulating volume.

- Haemorrhage.
- Gastrointestinal fluid loss.
- Burns.

2. Distributive. An increase in the volume of the circulatory system.

- Septicaemia.
- Anaphylaxis.
- Spinal cord injury.
- Anaesthesia.

3. Cardiogenic. Reduction in cardiac output secondary to pump failure.

- Myocardial infarction.
- Myocardial contusion.
- Arrhythmias.

4. Obstructive. Resistance to flow.

- Tension pneumothorax.
- Haemopneumothorax.
- Cardiac tamponade.
- Pulmonary embolism
- Flail chest.

5. Dissociative. Abnormal release of oxygen to the tissues.

- Anaemia.
- Carbon monoxide poisoning.
- Cyanide poisoning.

Phases of shock

Shock may be divided into three phases:

1. Compensated shock. Preservation of vital organ function by compensatory mechanisms. There is peripheral vasoconstriction including an increased heart rate, and water and salt re-absorption in the kidney. The clinical signs and symptoms are:

- Agitation/confusion.
- Tachycardia.
- Tachypnoea.
- Skin pallor.
- Decreased capillary return.
- Cold peripheries.
- Normal blood pressure.

2. Decompensated shock. Vital organ function is impaired and clinical deterioration progresses. The clinical signs and symptoms are:

- Falling blood pressure.
- Decreasing conscious level.
- Reduced or absent urine output.
- Kussmal breathing.

3. Irreversible shock. A terminal event, irreversible changes to vital organs. The diagnosis is retrospective and is based upon failure of a patient in decompensated shock to respond to appropriate treatment.

Hypovolaemic shock

Hypovolaemic shock is the commonest type of shock encountered in the trauma victim. It is divided into four categories in adults depending upon the magnitude of fluid loss.

1. Class I shock (up to 15% of circulating volume).
In the young healthy adult this class of shock may produce no obvious change in clinical signs or symptoms. In the absence of active fluid replacement compensatory mechanisms will restore circulating volume within 24 h.

2. Class II shock (15–30% circulating volume). In the healthy young adult this degree of hypovolaemia will produce changes in clinical signs including tachycardia, increase in respiratory rate, a thready pulse (decreased pulse pressure) and mild anxiety. Blood pressure is generally maintained within normal limits. Initial resuscitation is with crystalloid or colloid. Blood replacement may be required after the initial resuscitation phase to correct anaemia.

3. *Class III shock (30–40% circulating volume).* Patients with this degree of shock present with the classical picture of shock, marked tachycardia, hypotension, confusion, and pale sweaty extremities. Although initial management may be with crystalloid or colloid, blood transfusion is usually required to correct anaemia.

4. *Class IV shock (> 40% circulating volume).* Rapid loss of fluid to this degree may result in electro-mechanical dissociation (EMD) arrest and death unless immediate fluid replacement is initiated. The patient is confused or unconscious, blood pressure is low or unobtainable, surgical intervention may be required to control bleeding.

	Class I	Class II	Class III	Class IV
Blood loss (ml)[a]	Up to 750	750–1500	1500–2000	> 2000
Blood loss (% blood volume)	Up to 15%	15–30%	30–40%	> 40%
Pulse rate	< 100	> 100	> 120	> 140
Blood pressure	Normal	Normal	Decreased	Decreased
Pulse pressure	Normal or increased	Decreased	Decreased	Decreased
Respiratory rate	14–20	20-30	30–40	> 35
Urine output (ml/h)	> 30	20–30	5–15	Negligible
Mental state	Slight anxiety	Mild anxiety	Anxious, confused	Confused, lethargic
Fluid replacement	Crystalloid	Crystalloid	Crystalloid and blood	Crystalloid and blood

[a]Based on a 70 kg man.

This classification can be remembered using the scores of a game of tennis love (0)–15 (class I), 15–30 (class II), 30–40 (class III) and 40 plus.

Fluid therapy

Much controversy exists as to the type of fluid to be used in the initial resuscitation phase of hypovolaemic shock. Initially resuscitation will usually be carried out with either crystalloid (normal saline or Hartmann's) or colloid (haemaccel®, gelofusine or albumin). The type of fluid used is less important than the speed and rate of imitation of resuscitation.

Further reading

American College of Surgeons Committee on Trauma. In: *Advanced Trauma Life Support Program for Physicians*. Chicago: American College of Surgeons, 1993.

Related topics of interest

SHOULDER INJURIES

These injuries can be divided according to whether they affect soft tissues or soft tissues and bones. Shoulder injuries may also have a number of significant associated injuries, particularly of the brachial plexus, which can be missed if a thorough assessment is not undertaken.

Examination

Shoulder examination should commence with inspection, looking particularly for the bony contours, distortion of the soft-tissue mantle (by bone or bony spikes as a result of an underlying fracture or dislocation), deformity of the joint or its margins or lack of symmetry with the other shoulder.

Active and passive movements should be tested in all planes to the limits achievable by the patient. Careful assessment of the hand with respect to the blood supply and neurological abnormality should be performed. Each major nerve in the upper limb should be formally tested to exclude associated brachial plexus injuries.

Soft-tissue injuries

Apart from the frequent skin and superficial soft-tissue injuries to the shoulder which present so often to A&E Departments, there are a number of soft-tissue injuries specific to the shoulder.

Dislocation

Dislocation is by far the most common significant soft-tissue shoulder injury and it may be associated with bony injuries.

1. Anterior dislocation. This is the most common shoulder dislocation and commonly results from a fall producing external rotation of the shoulder. It occurs most commonly in the young adult and the elderly. Anterior dislocation of the humerus from the glenoid results in damage to the anterior structures of the shoulder joint.

The shoulder is extremely painful and the patient reluctant to allow it to be moved. On examination the acromium is prominent with an apparently concave contour to the lateral aspect of the upper arm. The humeral head may be palpable in the axilla. Plain radiography shows the characteristic appearance of anterior dislocation.

Treatment: reduction can be achieved by a number of methods, usually following the administration of an opiate analgesic with or without a benzodiazepine. Before reduction, sensation over the 'regimental badge' area (the outer aspect of the upper arm) which is supplied by the axillary (circumflex) nerve should be assessed as this is the most common neurological complication of dislocation.

- Kocher's method is the most common. Following traction to the arm with the elbow flexed, the arm is gradually externally rotated. The shoulder is then adducted and the elbow moves across the chest. Finally the shoulder is internally rotated. The method is repeated if initially unsuccessful.
- Hippocratic method: traction is applied to the arm and the humeral head eased back into place by a stockinged foot placed in the axilla.
- Gravitational traction: the patient lies face down with his arm hanging over the side of the couch, with muscle relaxation and analgesia the shoulder may spontaneously relocate over about an hour.

Following reduction the arm is held against the trunk in an appropriate sling or body bandage for about 4 weeks, in order to prevent external rotation and redislocation. More rapid mobilization is encouraged in the elderly in order to reduce the likelihood of joint stiffness. Recurrent dislocation is relatively common in younger patients.

Anterior dislocations of the shoulder occasionally present some days after occurrence. A general anaesthetic is usually required for reduction which may have to be carried out as an open procedure.

2. Posterior dislocation. This results from a fall on an outstretched internally rotated hand, direct trauma to the shoulder or, classically, from the jolt from an electric shock or during an epileptic fit.

The AP radiograph may well appear normal, or the so-called 'light-bulb' sign (rotation of the humeral head so that in outline it looks more symmetrical and like a light bulb than a walking stick) may be present. Diagnosis is confirmed by an axillary view.

Reduction is achieved by traction to the arm in 90° of abduction at the shoulder, followed by external rotation of the limb. Stable reductions are rested in a sling, unstable reductions in a shoulder spica.

3. Luxatio erecta. This rare dislocation presents with the arm held in abduction, often above the head. Reduction is achieved by applying traction to the arm as it lies then bringing the arm into adduction. Following reduction, the arm is immobilized as is an anterior dislocation.

4. Recurrent shoulder dislocation. This is relatively common, and consideration should be given to surgical repair of the damaged shoulder joint capsule.

Rotator cuff injuries

These injuries are particularly common in the elderly and characteristically produce a 'painful arc' syndrome with discomfort over an arc of abduction centred at 90° of abduction. Extensive tears may result in inability to abduct the arm more than a few degrees from the body. Initial treatment is with intensive physiotherapy, but surgery should be considered in selected patients if symptoms persist.

Frozen shoulder

This is a broad term loosely used to describe a number of conditions characterized by pain and restriction of movement. Occasionally secondary to trauma, it also occurs idiopathically. Invariably pain is severe with stiffness. When the pain resolves, the stiffness persists and an episode may take 18 months to 2 years to settle. Physiotherapy is especially beneficial once the pain begins to resolve.

Acromio-clavicular joint dislocation

These injuries are relatively common, particularly in sporting individuals who fall on to the shoulder. Local tenderness occurs over the lateral end of the clavicle, which is usually abnormally prominent. The diagnosis is confirmed by stress (weight bearing) views of *both* acromioclavicular joints, which will demonstrate joint widening on the affected side. If there is little or no instability, treatment is with a broad arm sling for 4–6 weeks. Gross instability (where all the scapulo-clavicular ligaments are ruptured) may require surgical repair.

Bony injuries

Fracture of the scapula

Rarely, the scapula may be fractured by a direct blow or by the patient falling on to, or being thrown on to, his scapula. These injuries may be accompanied by a large haematoma situated within the fascia surrounding the scapula. Treatment is by immobilization in a broad arm sling and analgesia. Complex scapula fractures may involve the gleno-humeral joint; conservative treatment is usually appropriate but occasionally open reduction and internal fixation will be required.

Fracture of the clavicle

Clavicular fractures are common and rarely require any other treatment than immobilization in a broad arm sling and analgesia. Occasionally there may be a wound over the clavicle, in which case the fracture is treated as a compound fracture with appropriate surgical debridement. Clavicular fractures should be checked for neurovascular damage to the hand. Care should be taken not to miss a sternoclavicular dislocation; if the clavicle dislocates posteriorly relative to the sternum, acute airway compromise may occur.

Coracoid fractures

Coracoid fractures are rare and usually result from direct trauma to the shoulder. Conservative treatment is usually appropriate.

Proximal humeral fractures

These fractures were classified by Neer into six groups, and usually result from direct trauma or a fall on an outstretched hand:

- Group I – fractures of all areas with no displacement or minimal displacement or angulation.
- Group II – fractures of the anatomical neck displaced by more than 1 cm.
- Group III – significantly displaced or angulated fractures of the surgical neck.
- Group IV – all fractures of the greater tuberosity.
- Group V – fractures of the lesser tuberosity.
- Group VI – fracture dislocations.

Group I and group II injuries are treated conservatively, initially in a collar and cuff. Immobilization is usually required for about 3–6 weeks. In the elderly, group III fractures (significantly displaced or angulated fractures of the surgical neck) usually settle with conservative treatment in a collar and cuff. In younger patients, manipulation under anaesthesia or open reduction and internal fixation may be necessary. Group IV and V fractures may be treated conservatively or surgically depending on the size and displacement of bony fragments. Group VI fracture dislocations are usually managed by closed reduction, although some may require fixation of bony fragments. An expert orthopaedic opinion should be sought.

| Investigation | Routine plain radiographs are the mainstay of investigation in shoulder injuries; however, if acute reconstruction of fractures or corrective surgery for soft-tissue injuries is contemplated, CT or MRI scanning may be necessary. |

Further reading

McRae R. *Practical Fracture Treatment*, 3rd Edn. Edinburgh: Churchill Livingstone, 1994.

Related topics of interest

Brachial plexus injuries (p. 46)
Elbow injuries: adults (p. 82)
Elbow injuries: children (p. 86)
Hand injuries (p. 116)
Injury patterns (p. 160)
Long bone fractures (p. 189)
Peripheral nerve injuries (p. 234)
Wrist injuries (p. 324)

SOFT-TISSUE INJURIES

Soft-tissue injuries comprise the majority of the 'minor injury' component of accident and emergency work. The initial priority is to exclude damage to underlying bone, nerves, vessels and tendons. The rationale behind the treatment of soft-tissue injuries can be best understood in the light of the physiological processes taking place during the healing process.

Wound healing

A soft-tissue injury involves the tearing of normal tissues, resulting in localized bleeding, with the release of histamine, bradykinin and serotonin from mast cells and platelets. The consequent vasodilatation and increased capillary permeability produce the classical signs of acute inflammation, namely, warmth, pain, swelling and loss or reduction in function. This acute inflammatory response begins within minutes of the injury and lasts for 3–4 days. Healing takes several weeks from the time of injury, the duration of the healing phase depending on the patient's age, severity and extent of the injury, co-existing diseases (diabetes, peripheral vascular disease) and the management of the injury.

Treatment of soft-tissue injuries

The acronym *'RICE' and 'analgesia'* summarize the specific components of early treatment.

Rest	During the first few days after injury, pain and swelling will restrict the degree of mobility. At this stage the early healing tissues will have little intrinsic mechanical strength and undue exertion may exacerbate the original injury.
Ice	Crushed ice or cold packs (frozen peas) wrapped in a towel to protect the skin from cold injury are applied for 10–15 min/hour for the first 2 days. This serves as local analgesia in addition to causing vasoconstriction, thus reducing oedema secondary to capillary leak. Longer exposure to cold will lead to a reactive vasoconstriction with exacerbation of symptoms. There is no benefit from application of ice packs after the first 48 hours.
Compression	Properly applied graduated compression bandages may reduce swelling by increasing interstitial tissue pressure. The commonly used tubular bandages rarely provide the correct degree of compression, but provide a feeling of support and are therefore of some psychological benefit.

Elevation	Elevation of the affected part above the level of the heart reduces oedema and pain.
Analgesia	An appropriate analgesic should be prescribed. In the absence of any contraindication, non-steroidal anti-inflammatory drugs are most appropriate as, in addition to their analgesic action, they reduce vasodilatation, capillary permeability and oedema.
Later treatment	After the first 48 hours, application of local heat is beneficial in that it leads to vasodilatation which promotes tissue healing. Gentle mobilization can usually begin at this stage. The majority of soft-tissue injuries settle satisfactorily with this regimen. In more severe injuries, those in athletes, the elderly or in those slow to respond to conservative management, referral for assessment and treatment by a physiotherapist is warranted.

Specific soft-tissue complications of injury

Myositis ossificans	Myositis ossificans (post-traumatic ossification) is a condition in which ossification of a haematoma, resulting from severe bony injury around a joint, occurs secondary to migration of osteoblasts from the disrupted periosteum. The condition is classically seen around the elbow joint following a supracondylar fracture. This complication is seen more commonly in children and in head injured patients. It may be prevented by immobilizing the joint to prevent or reduce haematoma formation. In severe cases excision of the bony mass may be warranted once the original injury has healed.
Sudeck's atrophy (reflex sympathetic dystrophy)	This is characterized by a painful, swollen, tender limb with a tense shiny appearance to the skin, loss of function of the affected part and, in extreme cases, atrophy of the hairs. Radiography reveals diffuse decalcification of the bones of the affected region. This condition may be seen as a complication of any injury, and is thought to be due to a defect in the sympathetic nervous system. The condition may gradually resolve of its own accord, although this can take up to 2 years. Physiotherapy is needed in the interim to maintain function. Guanethidine nerve blocks are sometimes of benefit. Referral to a pain clinic should be considered.

Degloving injury　　　　　Degloving injuries result from the application of shearing forces to the skin sufficient to shear the skin from its underlying connective tissue base and thus to remove its blood supply. The skin at initial presentation may look normal. The mechanism of injury should suggest the possibility of degloving injury, e.g. a car tyre running over the limb, a motorcyclist thrown from his cycle and planing down the road, or the classical injury of catching a wedding ring in the handle of a door, shearing the soft-tissues off in the process. All such cases should be referred for plastic surgical assessment. In the case of degloving injuries of the finger, amputation is usually required.

Further reading

English BK. Treatment and rehabilitation of soft-tissue injuries. *Surgery,* 1996; 226–8.

Related topics of interest

SPLENIC INJURIES

The spleen is the most common solid organ to be injured in blunt abdominal trauma. Seventy-five per cent of splenic injuries arise from blunt trauma, and of these, 50% are associated with other intra-abdominal injuries, 50% with other extra-abdominal injuries. The incidence of associated intra-abdominal injuries in penetrating splenic trauma is over 90%.

Splenic injuries may be graded from grade I (subcapsular haematoma less than 10% surface area, capsular tear less than 1 cm depth), to grade V (completely shattered spleen with devascularizing hilar injury).

Structure and function

The spleen, which is the largest single mass of lymphoid tissue in the body, has important immunological and reticuloendothelial functions, in particular the phagocytosis of encapsulated bacteria. Its long axis lies along the shaft of the tenth rib and it is surrounded by peritoneum which passes to the left kidney as the lienorenal ligament carrying the splenic vessels. The splenic artery, which runs along the upper border of the pancreas, divides into superior and inferior branches which, in turn, divide into end arteries. The end arteries run into splenic segments which are anatomically distinct and usually four in number (range 3–7).

Diagnosis and investigations

The mechanism of injury may give the first clue to the possibility of splenic trauma. It should be remembered that, for anatomical reasons, splenic injuries are associated with left lower rib fractures. Localized physical signs or the presence of an acute abdomen may suggest splenic injury, but physical examination may be completely normal.

Both diagnostic peritoneal lavage and ultrasound are effective in the investigation of splenic trauma, but the gold standard *if the patient is stable* is CT scanning, which is both sensitive and specific. It is important to recognize that in the unstable patient, the most important investigation is a laparotomy.

Splenectomy or no splenectomy?

Because of the splenic functions referred to above and the consequences of splenectomy, where possible splenic preservation is desirable, but not at the cost of immediate risk to the patient's life. If the patient is haemodynamically unstable, the correct treatment remains prompt laparotomy.

Preservation of the spleen can be achieved by 'conservative' surgery or by adopting a non-operative approach.

1. Indications for operative salvage. These include:

- haemodynamic stability (blood loss less than 500 ml);
- no coagulopathy;
- minimal /moderate splenic disruption;
- no hilar damage;
- minimal associated injuries.

In such cases it may be appropriate to attempt to save some or all of the spleen.

2. Non-operative management. Approximately one-third of patients with splenic injuries undergo splenectomy, and one-third some form of surgical salvage procedure. The remainder are treated conservatively. Injured spleens can heal spontaneously and a conservative approach has particularly been recommended in children in view of the risk of overwhelming post-splenectomy infection (OPSI).

3. Indications for conservative management. These include:

- haemodynamic stability;
- no serious associated intra-abdominal injuries;
- no significant extra-abdominal injuries;
- no hilar damage;
- no massive splenic disruption (on CT scanning).

Conservative management is not advocated in penetrating trauma nor in patients aged over 60. However, even if these criteria are strictly applied, approximately 15% of patients will subsequently require operative intervention.

Complications of splenic injury

The mortality of properly treated splenic injuries is low and death is usually the result of associated injuries, although it rises significantly in older patients to around 65%. As well as post-operative bleeding, complications include pneumonia, effusion, subphrenic abscess, and generalized sepsis.

Delayed splenic rupture may occur up to 2 weeks post-trauma due to rupture of a subcapsular haematoma, post-traumatic cyst or lysis of a clot. Some cases have been reported where the initial CT scan was normal.

Effects of splenectomy

Effects of splenectomy include:

- increased risk of sepsis;

- 30% more minor infections;
- increased platelet count;
- increased red cell count.

Following splenectomy, patients are less able to opsonize and phagocytose encapsulated organisms. The immunological effects of post-traumatic splenectomy are less severe than for elective splenectomy for non-trauma; this may be due to the preservation of implanted splenic fragments within the peritoneum.

The overwhelming post-splenectomy infection (OPSI) syndrome may occur immediately after splenectomy or years later. It commences with flu-like symptoms and progresses rapidly to DIC with hypoglycaemia and shock. The mortality is of the order of 50% and the risk of occurrence 2% in splenectomized children, 0.25% in adults. There is a decreased risk following anti-pneumococcal vaccination, but penicillin should be continued for at least 3 years following splenectomy.

Further reading

Mann C, Russell RCS, William N (eds). *Bailey and Love's Short Practice of Surgery,* 22nd Edn. London: Chapman & Hall, 1996.

Related topics of interest

SPLINTAGE

Musculoskeletal injuries are a significant cause of morbidity and mortality following trauma. Appropriate use of splintage will reduce the complications of major and minor bony injury.

When splinting a long-bone fracture, the joint above and the joint below should be immobilized. The pulse, circulation and sensation of the limb should be assessed before and after any movement of a fractured limb or reduction of a displaced fracture, as well as before and after the application of a splint. The circulation can be monitored using pulse oximetry.

Effects of splintage

Correct use of splintage reduces morbidity and mortality by the following means:

- Reduced blood loss. Traction in closed femoral fractures reduces blood loss in animal models by 20%.
- Reduction of the incidence of fat embolism.
- Reduction or prevention of neurovascular damage. Certain fractures and dislocations are particularly associated with such problems (e.g. displaced tibial fractures and vascular compromise or posterior hip dislocation and sciatic nerve damage).
- Prevention of skin problems. Ischaemic necrosis may be reduced or prevented by rapid reduction of displaced fractures or fracture dislocations.
- Reduction of pain. As well as making the patient more comfortable, reducing pain will improve the patient's cardiovascular status.
- Facilitation of patient handling, package and transportation.

Types of splintage

The following types of splintage are in common use:

1. Manual splintage. Manual stabilization of the cervical spine or of long-bone fractures is an appropriate initial method of immobilization.

2. Traction splintage. Traction allows gradual realignment of displaced bony fractures with relaxation of muscle in spasm. Manual traction can be followed by appropriate splintage, or a formal traction splint (Sager®, Donway® or Hare® splint) can be used. Traction splintage is ideal for lower limb, especially femoral, fractures. Pulling the femur out to length reduces the volume of the thigh and reduces the space available for internal haemorrhage.

3. *Triangular bandage and pads.* This is the ideal mode of immobilization in upper arm, forearm and elbow injuries. Triangular bandages applied as a narrow or broad band can be used to support lower-limb fractures.

4. *Frac straps*®. These velcro straps are used in a similar manner to rolled triangular bandages.

5. *Box splints.* The application of a box splint requires the limb to be straightened, and this may not always be possible in the pre-hospital environment without appropriate analgesia. However, box splints can provide appropriate immobilization in selected upper and lower limb fractures.

6. *Vacuum splints.* Vacuum splints are composed of a tough fabric shell (usually plastic) filled with synthetic beads. When the splint is formed around a limb and the air extracted using a hand or foot pump, a semi-rigid splint conforming to the enclosed limb is produced. These splints avoid the potential pressure problems associated with inflatable splints.

7. *Inflatable splints.* Inflatable splints were formerly in regular use, but it is now believed that the pressure exerted on the limb after the cylindrical splint has been inflated can cause pressure on the microcirculation and hence vascular compromise.

Recommended methods of splintage

1. *Cervical spine.* Manual immobilization then sandbags, collar and tape.

2. *Clavicle.* Broad arm sling.

3. *Sternoclavicular joint.* Broad arm sling.

4. *Acromioclavicular joint.* Broad arm sling.

5. *Upper limb.*

- Shoulder dislocation – patient's manual support with other arm.
- Fracture of neck of humerus – broad arm sling.

- Fracture of shaft of humerus – broad arm sling with folded triangular bandage above and below fracture.
- Supracondylar fracture of the humerus – padding and narrow triangular bandage to torso, or vacuum splint contoured to deformity.
- Dislocated elbow – as supracondylar fracture of humerus.
- Forearm fractures – padded box splint; if elbow flexed, broad arm sling.
- Wrist fractures – broad arm sling.

6. *Hip dislocation.* These are usually posterior, as the limb is characteristically flexed and internally rotated, splintage to the opposite limb with pads and triangular bandages is appropriate.

7. *Fractures of the pelvis.* The use of a vacuum mattress provides adequate splintage, although a reversed extrication device (KED® or RED®) can be used. The pneumatic antishock garment can be used to provide emergency splintage of pelvic fractures.

8. *Lower limb.*

- Neck of femur. Figure-of-eight bandage around the ankles and rolled triangular bandages around the legs (pad between the legs). Traction splintage will relieve pain and provides excellent immobilization.
- Fracture of shaft of femur. Reduce and apply a traction splint or, on arrival in hospital, a Thomas splint.
- Supracondylar fracture of femur. Padded box splint.
- Tibial plateau fracture. Padded box splint or equivalent.
- Patella dislocation. If unreduced, use padding and rolled triangular bandages; following reduction, consider the use of a box splint.
- Fracture of tibia and fibula. Realign and apply a long leg box splint or traction splint.
- Ipsilateral femoral and tibial fractures. Traction splintage.
- Ankle fractures. Early reduction followed by immobilization in a box splint is ideal; if delays are inevitable, consider a vacuum splint.

Further reading

Greaves I, Hodgetts T, Porter K. *Emergency Care: A Textbook for Paramedics.* London: WB Saunders, 1997.

Related topics of interest

SPORTS INJURIES

Sports injuries account for approximately 10% of A&E Department attendances. With the increasing promotion of sport and leisure activities, this figure is likely to increase .There is no such thing as an injury-free sport.

Classification

Sports injuries may be divided into:

- acute injuries; and
- chronic (overuse) injuries.

They may also be divided into:

- sports-specific injuries; and
- non-sports-specific injuries.

Non-sports-specific injuries (for example, ankle sprains) also occur in non-athletes; the majority of sports-specific injuries are chronic overuse injuries, although acute specific injuries do occur. Examples of sports-specific injuries include stress fractures, Achilles tendonitis and flexor tendon pulley injuries.

In general, sports injuries are perceived to be musculoskeletal injuries; however, it must not be forgotten that injuries from sport may be life-threatening, for example tension pneumothorax in crush injury due to a collapsing rugby scrum, cervical spine injury in equestrian accidents or airway obstruction following loss of consciousness in contact sports.

A return to sport in the unfit individual may precipitate medical problems, including cardiac arrest. Clinicians should always be mindful of the possibility of underlying illness such as diabetes.

Acute injuries

General principles

Acute injuries occur due to direct (for example, a kick to the quadriceps muscle) or indirect trauma (for example, bony avulsion due to muscle contracture of rectus femoris in posterior cruciate avulsion). Features of acute injury include:

- pain;
- tenderness;
- swelling;
- loss of function.

Treatment depends on

- nature of the injured tissue;
- magnitude of the injury;
- the patient's physical expectations.

Some injuries require mandatory surgical repair in order to return to high-level sport; however, the majority of sporting injuries can be managed conservatively. The principles of conservative management are:

> **R** – rest
> **I** – ice
> **C** – compression support
> **E** – elevation

usually in combination with analgesia and non-steroidal anti-inflammatory drugs.

Muscular injuries

Traumatic muscle rupture can be either complete or partial, the majority can be treated conservatively. The initial injury produces an inflammatory response which is followed by a phase of healing, repair and fibrosis.

Diffuse extensive muscle injury can be assessed accurately by ultrasound scanning. Localized collections of fluid can be aspirated under aseptic conditions using ultrasound guidance which enhances the quality of, and reduces the time to, recovery.

The majority of muscle ruptures (for example, long head of biceps or rectus femoris) require only conservative treatment. Rarely, surgical repair is necessary, for example in major quadriceps tears.

Physiotherapy is an important component of rehabilitation, preventing muscle contracture and shortening due to fibrosis with a consequent risk of chronic or recurrent injury. Specific advice on muscle stretching and warm-up regimes will help to prevent re-injury.

Tendon injuries

The majority of tendon injuries are closed injuries due to indirect forces producing partial or complete avulsions or ruptures. Occasionally penetrating injuries occur due to lacerations.

Complete tendon injuries are usually associated with little or no pain, whereas incomplete injuries may be extremely painful. Complete injuries are usually accompanied by loss of function.

1. Achilles tendon rupture. Rupture of the Achilles tendon is the most common tendon rupture, and patients frequently complain of a sensation similar to being kicked in the back of the leg. It is an injury which is unfortunately often missed on initial presentation to the A&E Department. For those who take part in sport at a high level, the best results in Achilles tendon rupture are achieved by surgical repair.

Partial tendon injuries and ruptures of non-essential tendons are treated conservatively.

Ligament injuries

Ligament injuries, like tendon injuries, are usually indirect, and similarly complete injuries tend to be painless whereas incomplete injuries are usually painful.

The ligament injury can occur in mid substance (for example, anterior cruciate injuries) or can occur as an avulsion with or without a bony fragment (for example, medial collateral ligament injury). Ligament injuries are graded:

- Grade I, some fibres torn, no laxity.
- Grade II, greater than 50% of fibres torn, with laxity.
- Grade III, complete tear with laxity.

Partial ligament injuries are treated conservatively. Complete injuries, such as of the medial collateral ligament, require surgical repair, post-operative splintage or protection and an appropriate physiotherapy regime. Mid-substance ruptures of the anterior cruciate ligament are irreparable and if the patient's physical requirements demand it, consideration should be given to reconstruction with a patellar tendon or hamstring graft.

Fibrocartilage injuries

The most common injury of this kind is to the menisci of the knee following a twisting injury on a semi-flexed knee. Swelling (effusion) is delayed. Displaced and unstable meniscal fragments require arthroscopic removal. The diagnosis is made on the initial history, and features include:

- swelling;
- locking;
- giving way.

Menisco-synovial detachments can be repaired, quite often these patients present with immediate swelling due to the development of a haemarthrosis from bleeding at the menisco-synovial junction.

Chronic injuries

General principles

Chronic injuries are overuse injuries due to repetitive activity. Examples include Achilles tendonitis and shin splints. Many problems occur because of inappropriate training objectives, inappropriate techniques and poor footwear. Treatment may therefore include:

- physiotherapy assessment and advice;
- modification of technique;
- modification or change of footwear;
- rest and immobilization, short term;
- non-steroidal anti-inflammatory drugs;
- steroid injections;
- surgical intervention.

The sooner a chronic injury is recognized and treated, the easier it is to rectify the clinical problem.

Muscular injuries

Recurrent muscle strains produce episodes of inflammation with scarring and muscle shortening. Appropriate massage, muscle stretching exercises and warm-up techniques will help to prevent a recurrence.

Tendon injuries

Chronic tendonitis occurs because of recurrent jarring of the tendon, producing pain, swelling and thickening. In older patients this may result in cyst formation and degeneration due to tendon microruptures.

Achilles and patellar tendonitis occur in part due to background biomechanical factors, especially hindfoot overpronation. Treatment should be aimed at the cause (sporting technique, orthotics) and local treatment measures (physiotherapy, steroid injection). Failure to settle with conservative measures is an indication for surgical decompression.

Tendon sheath injuries

Local tendon sheath swelling may occur on its own or in association with a tendonitis. Once a significant chronic problem is established, surgical decompression will be necessary.

Ligament injuries

Recurrent tears with scarring and swelling produce multiple lesions with calcification and ossification. The most commonly affected site is the ankle. Physiotherapy and attention to footwear may be of benefit.

Fibrocartilage injuries   As a result of recurrent shearing strains, small tears and cyst formation occur in the menisci. MRI investigation and arthroscopic examination is usually necessary.

Bone injuries   Overuse injury effecting the lower leg produces shin splints, one of the 'stress fractures'. Shin pain, tenderness, soreness and swelling are associated with physical activity. Locally there is bony tenderness due to periostitis and microfractures. Plain radiographs are often normal, the diagnosis is made on bone scan. Most overuse bony injuries are associated with underlying biomechanical problems. Once the acute symptoms have settled, the underlying problem should be dealt with using orthotics. Other areas commonly affected by stress fractures include the metatarsals.

Chronic compartment syndromes   Chronic compartment syndrome of the anterior compartment of the lower leg presents with shin pain during exercise which, unlike shin splints, stops in cessation of exercise. The diagnosis is confirmed by measurement of compartmental pressures during exercise. Fasciotomy will relieve the symptoms. Similarly, pain in the flexor compartment of the forearm occurs in motorcross sportsmen.

Sports injuries in children

Injuries to skeletally immature athletes are common, fortunately most do not have long-term implications. In particular, open epiphyses and apophyses are prone to injury in this population.

Examples of specific paediatric injuries include:

- Salter–Harris fractures due to falls.
- Tendon avulsions – the paediatric equivalent of tendon rupture. The tendon becomes detached with a fragment of bone.
- Traction apophysitis affecting the tibial tubercle (Osgood–Schlatter's disease) and the calcaneal apophysis (Sever's disease).

Further reading

Hutson MA. *Sports Injuries: Recognition and Management.* Oxford: Oxford University Press, 1996.

McLatchie GR. *Essentials of Sports Medicine.* Edinburgh: Churchill Livingstone, 1986.

Tubbs N. Sports injuries. In: *Cambridge Textbook of Accident and Emergency Medicine.* Cambridge: Cambridge University Press, 1997.

Related topics of interest

TETANUS AND GAS GANGRENE

Tetanus and gas gangrene are rare potentially life-threatening wound infections caused by a group of Gram-positive anaerobic bacilli, the *Clostridia*. (Q1) The *Clostridia* are spore producing organisms, the spores being widely distributed in nature, principally in soil and the human gut. The spores are resistant to heat and dessication. The effects of clostridial infections are due to the formation of exotoxins which produce the characteristic systemic effects of the infection. The incubation period is commonly 7–10 days, but may range from 4–21 days.

Tetanus

This infection of the central nervous system is due to the production of two exotoxins by the single organism *Clostridium tetani*:

1.   *Tetanospasmin.* A neurotoxin absorbed by motor nerve endings producing the characteristic muscular rigidity, spasms and convulsions associated with clinical tetanus.

2.   *Tetanolysin.* This causes haemolysis.

Tetanus is rare in the UK, there were 62 notifications between 1981–1986, three cases being in children under the age of 15, and 25 in persons over the age of 65. Elderly women form the highest risk group. In up to 50% of cases of clinical tetanus the wound acting as the nidus of infection is not evident: wounds as small as a thorn prick are known to have caused tetanus in the UK.

Although common in the environment and therefore a frequent wound contaminant, *C. tetanus* requires anaerobic conditions in which to reproduce. Adequate wound debridement and cleaning combined with tetanus prophylaxis is effective in preventing the condition.

Pathogenesis

The organism remains localized at the original entry wound. As the organism reproduces it releases exotoxin which passes centrally via motor nerve fibres. The toxin tetanospasmin blocks inhibitory impulses from presynaptic fibres in the anterior horn cells leading to motor hyperactivity and muscle spasticity. Four clinically distinct forms are recognized:

1. *Generalized tetanus.* This is by far the most common presentation. The clinical signs are:

- Dysphagia.
- Difficulty in chewing.
- Trismus (lock jaw): due to masseteric spasm.
- Risus sardonnicus: due to facial muscle spasm.
- Opisthotonos: hyperextension of the back, flexed adducted arms and extended legs.
- Generalized convulsions.

2. *Localized tetanus.* Spasm in muscles of the injured limb supplied by the same spinal segment as the affected area.

3. *Cephalic tetanus.* The least common form in which involvement is confined to the cranial nerves and follows localized injury to the head.

4. *Neonatal tetanus.* Common in the developing world, this is caused by the application of contaminated dung to the umbilical stump of the newborn. Mortality is 70%. It presents as irritability, facial grimacing and convulsions, commonly in the first week or 10 days after birth.

Diagnosis

Because the organism is localized to the original entry site, which may not be evident, isolation of the organism plays no part in the diagnosis, which is primarily clinical. Features which make the diagnosis of tetanus unlikely include:

- A definite history of immunization.
- Serum antitoxin levels > 0.01 units/ml.

Routine tetanus immunization was introduced in 1961, although those who served in the armed forces before this period are likely to have been immunized (this accounts for the fact that elderly women are the highest risk group).

Treatment

There are five components to the treatment of tetanus:

1. *Passive vaccination* with antitoxin to neutralize free toxin: 10 000 units of human tetanus immunoglobulin (HTI) by intravenous infusion (horse-derived immunoglobulin is not routinely used since the introduction of HTI because of the frequency of side effects).

2. *Primary vaccination* with tetanus toxoid. Infection does not confer immunity from infection.

3. *Antibiotics* to treat the localized infection of *C. tetani*. Use benzylpenicillin and metronidazole, or erythromycin if the patient is penicillin sensitive.

4. *Debridement* and cleaning the wound to remove the anaerobic environment conducive to growth of the organism.

5. *Medical and nursing care* on an ITU including, where necessary, paralysis, mechanical ventilation and total parenteral nutrition (patients are usually hypercatabolic).

Prognosis

In developed countries with full access to ITU the mortality is about 10%. Causes of death include:

- Respiratory failure.
- Pneumonia.
- Septicaemia.
- Multi-organ failure.

Prevention of tetanus

The components of prevention are primary vaccination and proper wound management.

1. *Primary vaccination.* The cornerstone of tetanus prevention is an active programme of primary immunization. The current recommendations in the UK are for primary vaccination with adsorbed tetanus toxoid (0.5 ml):

- Aged 3 months	First dose.
- 6–8 weeks after first dose	Second dose.
- 4–6 months after second dose	Third dose.
- Aged 5 years	First booster dose.
- Aged 15 years	Second booster dose.

Further booster doses are not recommended more frequently than every 10 years unless there is a definite indication because allergic reactions are more common.

2. *Proper wound management.*

- Surgical debridement: Removes devitalized tissue and foreign matter.
- Wound cleansing: Removes residual bacteria.
- Antibiotics: (if indicated) To kill residual bacteria.
- Immunization: See table below for recommendations. Dose of tetanus toxoid 0.5 ml IM/sec. Dose of anti-tetanus immunoglobulin 250–500 units IM.

It must be emphasized that antibiotics are no substitute for thorough debridement and cleansing.

History of toxoid vaccination	Clean minor wounds		Tetanus prone wounds	
	Toxoid	Immunoglobulin	Toxoid	Immunoglobulin
Unknown or less than three doses or more than 10 years since last dose	Yes	No	Yes	Yes
At least three doses	No	No	No	No

Factors determining tetanus proneness of wounds are:

- Any wound or burn more than 6 hours old.
- Any wound or burn which at any time after injury shows one or more of the following:
  (a) Significant degree of devitalized tissue.
  (b) Puncture wound.
  (c) Direct contact with soil or material likely to be contaminated with tetanus.
  (d) Clinical evidence of sepsis.

Gas gangrene

This infection is caused by the combined effects of several clostridial species:

- *C. perfringens* (*C. welchii*).
- *C. novyi.*
- *C. septicum.*

The exotoxins produced by these three organisms produce tissue necrosis, the necrotic tissue is broken down by:

- *C. sporonges.*
- *C. histiolyticum.*

Stages in the development of gas gangrene

- Necrosis of muscle tissue.
- Production of odourless gases (hydrogen and carbon dioxide).
- Breakdown of tissue barriers (endomysium and perimysium) by the enzymes hyaluronidase and collaginase, and local invasion of adjacent tissues by the infecting organisms.
- Increased tissue pressure (due to gas and necrotic tissue) leading to increased tissue necrosis.
- Putrefaction caused by *C. sporonges* and histiolyticum leading to gangrene and production of the characteristic odour.
- Toxaemia due to circulating exotoxins (not in the early stages of the process to circulating organisms).

Death rapidly ensues once toxaemia develops. In the early stages before putrefaction occurs the muscle has a characteristic brick-red colour. Once putrefaction ensues the muscle changes to a greenish-black colour before liquefaction occurs.

Treatment

There are four components to the treatment of gas gangrene:

1. Prophylaxis in high risk cases (e.g. contaminated wounds, high lower-limb amputations). Use benzylpenicillin or metronidazole.

2. Adequate wound toilet combined with wide debridement of all affected muscle.

3. Polyvalent antiserum against the three main exotoxins produced.

4. Hyperbaric oxygen. Failure to achieve adequate, early, wide debridement of infected tissue is probably the most common cause of failure to control gas gangrene in contaminated wounds.

Further reading

Immunisation Against Infectious Disease. London: HMSO, 1996.

Related topics of interest

Antibiotic therapy (p. 36)
Hepatitis B (p. 130)
Hepatitis C (p. 134)
HIV infection (p. 143)

THORACIC AND LUMBAR EPIDURAL ANAESTHESIA

Local anaesthetics introduced into the thoracic or lumbar epidural space are effective for either traumatic or surgical pain from the chest, abdomen, pelvis and lower limbs. An epidural catheter is usually inserted, allowing repeated doses or infusions to be given. Opiates may be added to the local anaesthetic for optimal effect. Epidural analgesia is particularly useful in:

- Chest or upper abdominal conditions (e.g. flail chest) which may impair deep breathing and coughing, leading to chest complications.
- Multiple injuries of the trunk and lower limbs.

Special training and skill is needed for insertion. Because of serious side-effects, patients should ideally be managed in a high-dependency area.

Advantages	• Complete analgesia is usually possible.
	• Analgesia may be maintained for several days, by a continuous infusion or repeated doses.
	• Surgery under epidural is possible with appropriate 'topping up'.
	• Lack of sedation (with local anaesthetics, although epidural opiates may cause drowsiness).
	• Chest complications may be reduced, by allowing painless deep breathing and coughing.
	• May reduce the metabolic and hormonal stress response to trauma and surgery.
	• Possible protection against deep venous thrombosis.
Complications	*1. Common.*
	• Hypotension, due to sympathetic blockade (severe in hypovolaemia). Sympathetic vasoconstrictor nerves arise from spinal cord segments T1–L1/2, and cardiac sympathetic fibres from T1–4. The intercostal and, in severe cases, the phrenic nerves (C3–C5) may also be affected.
	• Muscle weakness (minimized by using dilute local anaesthetic solutions).
	• Urinary retention.
	• Pruritus, sedation and nausea (epidural opiate side-effects).

2. *Uncommon/rare.*

- Inadvertent dural puncture ($\approx$ 1%), with CSF leak and headache.
- Local anaesthetic toxicity (see Local blocks: regional anaesthesia), from absolute overdose or injection into an epidural vein.
- Epidural haematoma with spinal cord compression in patients with coagulopathy (e.g. in major haemorrhage).
- Excessively high segmental block with hypotension, bradycardia and impaired ventilation (see above).
- 'Total spinal' anaesthetic from unrecognized intrathecal injection, with unconsciousness, severe hypotension and apnoea.
- Infection (epidural abscess, meningitis).
- Permanent neurological deficit (extremely rare).

Contraindications

1. Absolute.

- Coagulopathy (therefore unsuitable in the acute phase of major trauma).
- Sepsis at insertion site.

2. Relative.

- Impaired cardiac output, such as aortic stenosis, hypovolaemia (uncompensated vasodilation may cause catastrophic hypotension).
- Neurological deficit and spinal injury (mainly a medico–legal contraindication).
- Treatment with aspirin or sub-cutaneous heparin (controversial).
- Septicaemia (risk of blood-borne epidural infection).

Practical management

1. An anaesthetist must insert the epidural, give the first dose and be available at all times while the epidural is in use.

2. Resuscitation facilities must be available.

3. A large-bore cannula must be in place at all times, to allow rapid fluid infusion if hypotension occurs.

4. Monitor the following frequently during epidural infusion:

- Pulse rate.
- Blood pressure.
- Respiratory rate (if opiates are used).
- Level of block (by skin dermatome testing).

5. *Treatment of epidural-induced hypotension:*

- Oxygen (if severe).
- Rapid IV fluids.
- Stop epidural infusion.
- Ephedrine increments 3–5 mg IV (if severe).
- Contact anaesthetist.
- Exclude other causes (e.g. occult bleeding).

6. *Treatment of respiratory depression:*

- Oxygen.
- Assist ventilation if necessary.
- Stop epidural infusion.
- Contact anaesthetist.
- Consider IV naloxone if opiates are used.

Further reading

Löfström JB, Bengtsson M. Spinal and extradural analgesia. In: Nunn JF, Utting JE, Brown BR Jr. (eds). *General Anaesthesia*, 5th Edn. London: Butterworths, 1989; 1086–105.

Puke M *et al.* Complications of regional analgesia. In: Nunn JF, Utting JE, Brown BR Jr. (eds). *General Anaesthesia*, 5th Edn. London: Butterworths, 1989; 1106–12.

Related topics of interest

THORACIC TRAUMA

Thoracic trauma remains a significant cause of preventable death in those patients reaching hospital alive following major trauma. The principal causes of death are hypoxia, hypercarbia and respiratory and metabolic acidosis, resulting from airway compromise, inadequate ventilation and/or lung perfusion and hypovolaemic shock.

Approximately 10% of those with blunt thoracic trauma require surgical intervention. Up to 30% of those with penetrating trauma require surgical intervention. The majority of thoracic trauma cases in the UK can be managed by adequate resuscitation and the judicious placing of a chest drain/drains by a competent doctor.

Life-threatening chest injuries

There are six immediately life-threatening chest injuries, all of which may be easily identified in the primary survey:

- Airway obstruction.
- Tension pneumothorax.
- Open pneumothorax.
- Massive haemothorax.
- Flail chest.
- Cardiac tamponade.

There are six potentially life-threatening chest injuries which should be identified during the secondary survey:

- Pulmonary contusion.
- Myocardial contusion.
- Aortic rupture.
- Diaphragmatic rupture.
- Tracheobronchial tree disruption.
- Oesophageal injury.

Injuries identified in the primary survey

1. Airway obstruction.
Diagnostic features:

- Agitation.
- Reduced conscious level.
- Cyanosis.
- Intercostal or subcostal retraction.
- Use of accessory muscles.
- Noisy breathing (stridor, gurgling, snoring).
- Decreased tidal volume.

Treatment:

- Maintain in-line cervical spine immobilization.
- High flow O_2.

- Simple airway manoeuvres (chin lift, head tilt or jaw thrust — caution in cervical spine injury).
- Airway adjuncts (oropharyngeal or nasopharyngeal airway).
- Endotracheal or nasotracheal intubation.
- Cricothyroidotomy.
- Surgical airway.

2.   Tension pneumothorax. Entry of air into one side of the pleural cavity through a one-way valve mechanism leads to unilateral increase in intrathoracic pressure and collapse of the ipsilateral lung, shift of the mediastinum away from the side of the air leak and consequent reduction in venous return and compression of the contralateral lung. The diagnosis is clinical, radiographic confirmation should not be awaited prior to treatment.

Diagnostic features (relate to the affected side unless indicated):

- Decreased chest movements.
- Decreased air entry.
- Hyper-resonant to percussion.
- Tracheal deviation away from the affected side.
- Shock.
- Cyanosis (late).
- Bradycardia (late).

Treatment:

- Initial: Needle thoracostomy through the second intercostal space in the mid-clavicular line.
- Definitive: Chest tube drainage.

Left-sided tension pneumothorax may mimic cardiac tamponade. Tension pneumothorax is commoner and is characterized by hyper-resonance to percussion on the affected side.

3.   Open pneumothorax. A defect in the chest wall as little as two-thirds the diameter of the trachea leads to preferential entry of air through the defect on inspiration, causing a 'sucking' wound, resulting in reduced ventilation and hypoxia.

Diagnostic features:

- Respiratory distress.
- A defect in the chest wall.

The diagnosis may be missed in the case of a posterior defect unless the patient is log rolled.

Treatment:

- Initial: place an occlusive dressing over the defect, one side being left open to prevent the formation of a tension pneumothorax.
- Definitive: insertion of a chest drain until surgical closure can be achieved.

4. *Massive haemothorax.* Rapid accumulation of more than 1500 ml of blood in the chest cavity. Lung collapse leads to hypoxia complicated by shock.

Diagnostic features:

- Shock.
- Decreased breath sounds on the affected side.
- Dullness to percussion on the affected side.

Treatment:

- Initial: fluid resuscitation, chest tube insertion.
- Definitive: thoracotomy if there is an initial drainage of 1500 ml of blood or continued loss of 200 ml per hour.

5. *Flail chest.* This is the presence of a segment of the chest wall with no bony continuity with the rest of the thoracic cage. Paradoxical movement of the flail segment combined with underlying lung contusion leads to hypoventilation, hypoxia and pulmonary shunting. The principal cause of the problems is the pulmonary contusion rather than the paradoxical movement of the flail segment.

Diagnostic features:

- Abnormally mobile segment on palpation.
- Crepitus on palpation.
- Paradoxical movement of the chest wall (may not be present initially due to chest wall splinting).

Treatment:

- Initial: adequate ventilation, supplemental oxygen, judicious fluid resuscitation (care should be taken not to over resuscitate in order to reduce the risk of ARDS).
- Definitive: mechanical ventilation, thoracic epidural.

6. *Cardiac tamponade.* Caused by blunt or penetrating trauma resulting in leakage of blood into the relatively undistensible pericardial sac which creates restricted cardiac filling. As little as 20 ml can cause significant clinical signs.

Diagnostic features:

- Becks triad (not always present): elevated venous pressure, decreased arterial pressure, muffled heart sounds.
- Pulsus paradoxus.
- Distended neck veins may be absent in the presence of hypovolaemia.

Treatment:

- Initial: fluid resuscitation (which leads to a temporary improvement in cardiac output), needle pericardiocentesis.
- Definitive: thoracotomy.

A left-sided tension pneumothorax can mimic cardiac tamponade and is more common. The presence of an EMD arrest in the absence of tension pneumothorax and hypovolaemia suggests the diagnosis of cardiac tamponade. Echocardiography will confirm the diagnosis.

Injuries identified in the secondary survey

1. *Pulmonary contusion.* This is the most common, potentially lethal chest condition in trauma, it causes delayed death by progressive respiratory failure. Careful monitoring of those with chest trauma is therefore required.

Diagnostic features:

- Hypoxia.
- Diffuse shadowing on chest X-ray.

Treatment:

- Initial: high flow oxygen.
- Definitive: intubation and ventilation.

2.   *Myocardial contusion.* The diagnosis is often missed or delayed.

Diagnostic features:

- Arrhythmias.
- Myocardial ischaemia/infarction.
- Ventricular dysfunction on echocardiography.

Treatment:
There is no specific treatment, arrhythmias are treated as appropriate. Patients with myocardial contusion are at risk of sudden death and should be monitored in an intensive care unit (ICU) or coronary care unit (CCU).

3.   *Aortic rupture.* Commonly fatal at the scene, such injuries result from road-traffic accidents or falls from a height. A partial tear may occur at the level of the ligamentum arteriosum an intact layer of adventitia containing the resultant haematoma.

Diagnostic features: abnormalities on CXR including:

- Widened mediastinum.
- Obliteration of the aortic knob.
- Deviation of the trachea to the right.
- Presence of a pleural cap.
- Elevation and rightward shift of the right mainstem bronchus.
- Depression of the left mainstem bronchus.
- Obliteration of the space between the pulmonary artery and the aorta.
- Deviation of the oesophagus (nasogastric) to the right.

No single sign is diagnostic, a widened mediastinum is the most consistent finding. The aortogram will be positive in 10% of cases when used liberally. Transoesophageal doppler or CT scan may be of use if available.

Treatment: Surgical repair or excision and grafting.

Left untreated the mortality from aortic rupture is said to be 50% per day.

4. *Diaphragmatic rupture.* Frequently missed, ruptured diaphragm occurs more commonly on the left than the right side where the liver obliterates the defect. Penetrating injuries cause small lacerations that develop over a period of time into a full hernia, right-sided hernias similarly present late.

Diagnostic features:

- The presence of a nasogastric tube or abdominal contents in the thorax on CXR.
- Presence of peritoneal lavage fluid flowing from a chest drain.

Although a left-sided rupture will show on a standard CXR, it may be mistaken for one of the following:

- Elevated left hemidiaphragm.
- Acute gastric dilatation.
- Loculated haemopneumothorax.
- Subpulmonary haematoma.

Treatment: Surgical repair.

5. *Tracheobronchial tree disruption.* Frequently fatal, tracheobronchial tree disruption may be caused by blunt or penetrating trauma.

Diagnostic features:

- Laryngeal disruption: hoarseness, subcutaneous emphysema, crepitus.
- Tracheal disruption: signs of airway obstruction, subcutaneous emphysema.
- Bronchial tree disruption: haemoptysis, subcutaneous emphysema, tension pneumothorax, persistent large air leak after chest drain insertion.

Treatment : Surgical repair.

6. *Oesophageal injury.* Almost always a result of penetrating injury, it may rarely be caused by a blow to the upper abdomen forcefully expelling the stomach contents and leading to linear tears in the lower oesophagus.

Diagnostic features:

- The presence of a left pneumothorax or haemothorax in the absence of rib fractures.

- A history of a blow to the upper abdomen or lower sternum in the presence of pain or shock out of proportion to the injury.
- The presence of particulate matter in the chest drain after blood has cleared.
- The presence of mediastinal air.

Treatment : Surgical repair.

Other manifestations of thoracic trauma

1. Subcutaneous emphysema. Characterized by subcutaneous crepitus. Although dramatic in appearance it requires no specific treatment other than treatment of the underlying cause.

2. Traumatic asphyxia. Petechial haemorrhage and plethora in the distribution of the superior vena cava secondary to its compression. Cerebral oedeama may occur. Treatment is that of the underlying injuries.

3. Simple pneumothorax. Chest tube drainage is the traditional treatment for traumatic simple pneumothorax. High-altitude air travel and positive pressure ventilation can convert an undrained simple pneumothorax into a tension pneumothorax.

4. Haemothorax. Drainage by chest tube is undertaken to prevent clotted haemothorax. Surgical intervention is not usually required.

5. Rib fracture.

- Ribs 1–3 and scapula: associated with major injury to head, neck spinal cord and great vessels with a mortality of 50%.
- Ribs 4–9: usually result in pneumothorax, haemothorax or pulmonary contusion.
- Ribs 10–12: associated with injury to the liver and spleen.

Adequate analgesia is required (oral analgesics, intercostal block, thoracic epidural) to allow adequate ventilation and prevent complications of collapse and pneumonia. Strapping of the chest wall is contraindicated.

6. Emergency thoracotomy. Emergency thoracotomy is rarely of benefit in victims of blunt trauma who have arrested. The outcome in victims of penetrating trauma with an EMD arrest due to cardiac tamponade or hypovolaemia is more promising if the arrest is recent or witnessed. A left thoracotomy is performed with internal cardiac massage and volume replacement. Cross clamping of the descending aorta with or without pericardiotomy is performed.

Further reading

American College of Surgeons Committee on Trauma. Abdominal trauma. In: *Advanced Trauma Life Support: Program for Physicians*. Chicago: American College of Surgeons, 1993; 141–58.

Robertson C, Redmond AD. *The Management of Major Trauma*. Oxford Handbooks in Emergency Medicine. Oxford: Oxford University Press, 1991.

Skinner D, Driscoll P, Earlam R. *ABC of Major Trauma*. London: BMJ Publications,1991; 46-50.

Related topics of interest

TOURNIQUETS

Tourniquets may be life saving in the pre-hospital environment to control external haemorrhage uncontrollable by other means such as external pressure, elevation and pressure points. They may be of value in the A&E Department to control catastrophic limb bleeding, and are routinely used in limb surgery to produce an exsanguinated field.

Safety

Safe practice recommendations for cuff pressure and duration of application are:

	Maximum cuff pressure	Maximum ischaemic time
Upper limb	200 mmHg	90 min
Lower limb	300 mmHg	120 min

Safe application involves using a wide cuff at the lowest possible pressure (100–150 mmHg above systolic pressure for the lower limb). Double cuffs reduce complications. Nerve lesions complicate the use of a correctly applied tourniquet in between 1 in 5000 and 1 in 8000 cases. Electromyographic studies have revealed abnormalities after as little as 20 minutes of application. Up to 70% of patients demonstrate electromyographic abnormalities without clinical symptoms following routine tourniquet use. Tourniquets may be reinflated following a 5 minute 'rest period' after 90 mins of inflation.

Previous femoro-popliteal bypass is an absolute contraindication to the application of a lower limb tourniquet.

Emergency use

If applied in the pre-hospital environment, a tourniquet should be released for 1 min every 15 mins. If it should remain in use after 60 mins, it should remain inflated thereafter without breaks in view of the potentially lethal effects of the release of cardiotoxic substances.

Related topics of interest

Amputation: traumatic (p. 18)
Compartment syndrome (p. 70)
Crush syndrome (p. 74)

TRAUMA SCORING

Trauma scoring allows the doctor to predict the likely outcome of a patient's injuries, it has two roles; to allow retrospective study of the outcome of trauma and trauma care, and to allow triage of trauma patients to appropriate medical facilities. This second role is more important if different levels of trauma facilities are available. A major role of trauma scoring in the UK is to establish through the major trauma outcome study (MTOS) whether trauma patients would benefit from the establishment of trauma centres.

Scoring systems

Psychological scoring systems

1. The trauma score (TS) (H. Champion, 1981) using the parameters: respiratory rate, respiratory effort, systolic BP, capillary refill time and the Glasgow coma scale (GCS). Probability of survival (Ps) was found to fall from 99% with a maximum trauma score of 16–0% with a score of 2.

2. The revised trauma score (RTS) (H. Champion, 1989). Eliminated respiratory effort and capillary refill time from the analysis. The RTS is therefore based on GCS, systolic BP and respiratory rate.

The trauma score and revised trauma score are physiological scoring systems. Anatomical scoring systems are available and are combined with physiological systems in *TR*auma score *I*njury *S*everity *S*core (TRISS) methodology. In the revised trauma score each parameter is scored as follows:

Respiratory rate	10–29	4
	> 29	3
	6–9	2
	1–5	1
	0	0
	0	0
Systolic BP	> 90	4
	76–89	3
	50–75	2
	1–49	1
	0	0

Glasgow Coma Scale	13–15	4
	9–2	3
	6–8	2
	4–5	1
	3	0

The relative importance of each factor is taken into account by multiplying each score by a weighting coefficient.

Glasgow Coma Scale	0.9368.
Systolic BP	0.7326.
Respiratory rate	0.2908.

The sum of the weighted values is the RTS and is related to the Ps as follows:

RTS (rounded to the nearest whole number)	Ps (%)
8	99
7	97
6	92
5	81
4	61
3	36
2	17
1	7
0	3

NB. The range of unrounded RTS scores is 7.84–0.

3. *The triage revised trauma score (TRTS)*. Because of the complexity of the RTS, a modification, the TRTS, has been proposed as a tool for triaging trauma patients. The TRTS, is the sum of the unweighted scores of the RTS: the maximum TRTS being 12, the minimum 0. In the USA a score of 3 or less in any one parameter (e.g. a total score of 11 or less) indicates the need for transfer to a level 1 trauma centre. The relationship between TRTS and Ps is as follows:

TRTS	Ps (%)
12	99.5
11	96.9
10	87.9
9	70.65
8	66.7
7	63.6
6	63.0
5	45.5
4	33.3
3	30.3
2	28.6
1	25.0
0	3.7

Problems with physiological trauma scoring

- Lack of experience amongst clinicians.
- Lack of validation for the very young or very old.
- Underscoring on initial assessment, due in part to assessment before physiological compensation has failed.

Anatomical scoring systems

Trauma may also be scored using anatomical systems (the injury severity scale, ISS), and anatomical and physiological methods are combined in TRISS methodology. Anatomical scoring is based on the abbreviated injury scale (AIS):

- Each injury is scored from 1 (minor) to 6 (untreatable) using standard lists of injuries.
- The ISS is calculated from the AIS. The ISS is the sum of the squares of the highest AIS scores from three of six predetermined body areas.
- An AIS score of 6 is untreatable and awarded a score of 75.
- A score of > 16 is considered to indicate major trauma.

An example of an ISS calculation

Region	Injury	AIS	AIS
Head/neck	Unconscious at scene	3	
	Basal skull fracture	4	16
	Occipital laceration	1	
Face	Fracture orbital floor	2	
Chest	Fractured ribs x2	4	16
	Bilateral haemothorax		
Extremities	Open fracture tibia	3	
Abdomen	Retroperitoneal		
	haemorrhage	3	9
	L2/3 spine abrasion	1	
External	Multiple abrasions	1	
	ISS = 9 + 16 + 16 = 41		

Reproduced with permission from BASICS Monographs on Immediate Care No. 9, *Trauma Scoring,* BASICS, 1993

TRISS methodology

TRISS methodology combines physiological (RTS) and anatomical (ISS) methods together with the age of the patient and the method of injury (blunt or penetrating). The Ps is defined as follows:

$$\frac{Ps}{1 + e^{-b}}$$

where $b = b_0 + b_1 (RTS) + b_2 (ISS) + b_3 (A)$

b_{0-3}: weighted coefficients based on American trauma data and different for blunt and penetrating trauma. A: age (score 0 if < 54, 1 if > 55).

TRISS methodology originally used data derived from American series, coefficients based on British data are now available.

- *M statistic*. Calculation of the M statistic is used to decide whether comparison between a study survival rate and the American database is valid. The M statistic has a value between 0 and 1, values less than 0.88 indicate that comparison of data would be invalid.

- *Z statistic*. The Z statistic is used to compare the outcome of trauma care systems between two groups of patients and hence between two hospitals:

$$Z = \frac{\text{number of survivors} - \text{predicted number of survivors}}{\int \text{sum of } [Ps - (1-Ps)]}$$

The normal range for Z is between −1.96 and +1.96. Z statistics are not valid unless the M statistic indicates that the groups are comparable with the American database.

Computer programmes are available for the calculation of TRISS methodology.

Further reading

Driscoll PA, Gurinnutt CL, Jimmerson CLeD, Goodall O (eds). *Trauma Resuscitation: the Team Approach*, London: Macmillan, 1993.

Hodgetts TJ, Davies S. *Trauma Scoring*. BASICS Monograph No 9. Ipswich: BASICS, 1993.

Related topics of interest

TRAUMA TEAMS

Improved trauma outcomes have been demonstrated in the USA following the introduction of regional and tertiary trauma centres. An important component of this form of trauma management is the trauma team. Evidence from the USA has demonstrated an improved outcome for patients with ISS greater than 12 if managed by organized teams rather than individual specialists on an *ad hoc* basis. With the dissemination of ATLS principles, hospitals in the UK are under increasing pressure to establish such teams. Where such teams have been introduced, there is already evidence of improved patient care.

Trauma teams in the UK

A recent study of 185 UK A&E Departments demonstrated that 61% had an effective trauma team or equivalent arrangement. The presence of a trauma team was not influenced by the number of A&E attendances or the staffing of the A&E Department.

Composition of the trauma team

Ideally, the team should be led by a consultant, indeed evidence now exists to suggest that senior team leadership is associated with lower mortality rates. It is clear that it is the experience and training of the team leader rather than his speciality that is important in improving outcome. Lack of senior team leadership is a particular problem in the UK, where a recent study found that a senior house officer was in charge of initial resuscitation in 57% of patients with an injury severity score of 16 or greater.

Ideally the trauma team should contain:

- doctor team leader (usually an A&E consultant);
- A&E medical staff;
- anaesthetist;
- orthopaedic surgeon;
- general surgeon;
- nursing staff [usually A&E-based, and ideally Advanced Trauma Nursing Certificate (ATNC) trained].

Clearly, the precise composition of a team will depend on the manpower and specialities available in any particular hospital.

The trauma team should be available 24 hours a day. Manpower constraints are unlikely, in the majority of centres in the UK, to allow around the clock resident consultant cover in A&E or in any other speciality.

Objectives of the trauma team	• To provide appropriate, experienced team leadership. • To ensure the presence of appropriately trained medical (ATLS) and nursing (ATNC) staff. • To provide stabilization and thorough assessment of the injured patient, using an established framework • To establish treatment priorities. • To reduce patient morbidity and mortality.

Costs

Since the main changes in establishing a trauma team are organizational, the principal costs involved are for education. With ATLS becoming an increasingly common requirement for career progression, the specific costs of trauma teams are likely to lessen.

Why are trauma teams effective?

Comparing care before and after the introduction of trauma teams, Driscoll and Vincent (1992) found significant reductions in the times taken for all aspects of resuscitation, except patient examination, even taking into account some variability in injury pattern and trauma team composition. The average time for resuscitation was reduced from 122 to 56 minutes. This change is clearly due to the ability of an integrated team to carry out tasks simultaneously.

The second advantage of the trauma team is the ability of a single team leader to establish clinical priorities and plan management accordingly.

Further reading

Dean GA, *et al.* The hospital trauma team: a model for trauma management. *Injury,* 1990; **21:** 68–70.

Driscoll PA, Vincent CA. Variations in trauma resuscitation and its effect on patient outcome. *Injury,* 1992; **23:** 111–15.

Kayemi AR, Nayeem N. The existence and composition of trauma teams in the UK. *Injury,* 1997; **28:** 119–21.

Yates DW, *et al.* Preliminary analysis of the care of injured patients in 33 British hospitals: first report of the United Kingdom Major Trauma Outcome Study. *British Medical Journal,* 1992; **305:** 737–40.

Related topics of interest

Advanced Trauma Life Support (ATLS) (p. 11)
United Kingdom trauma outcomes (p. 315)

TRIAGE

The term triage is derived from the French 'trier' to sort (not triager). The term appears to have been borrowed from the process of sorting coffee beans and was first used in a medical context by Baron Dominique Jean Larrey, chief surgeon to Napoleon Bonaparte. Triage on arrival is now required of A&E Departments by the Patient's Charter. Triage is a dynamic process and may need to be repeated as the patient's circumstances, situation or condition change.

The sorting of patients into priority groups prior to treatment will be required in two situations:

- Where the number of patients and the severity of their injuries does not exceed the available medical resources but it is necessary to select the more seriously injured for priority treatment. This is the situation in the average A&E Department.
- Where the number of patients and the severity of their injuries exceeds the available medical resources and it is necessary to identify those who will be given the best chance of survival with the most 'economical' use of time.

Triage categories

The commonly used triage categories (P system, T system and colour coding) are given in the following table:

Colour	P	T	Description
Red	P1	T1	Immediate
Yellow	P2	T2	Urgent
Green	P3	T3	Delayed
Blue*	–	T4	Expectant
White	Dead	Dead	Dead

*Green with folded corners revealing red, using the Cambridge cruciform card.

1. *Immediate.* (P1/T1) patients colour coded red are those in need of immediate medical attention.

2. *Urgent.* (P2/T2) patients colour coded yellow are considered to be those requiring treatment within 4–6 hours.

3. *Delayed.* (P3/T3) patients colour coded green do not require treatment within 6 hours.

4. *Expectant.* (T4) is used to identify those patients whose condition is so severe that the effort required to attempt to save them would compromise the survival of larger numbers of less seriously injured patients.

There is no 'P' equivalent to T4 although the armed forces use the term 'P1 hold'. This term should not be used in the civilian environment where the T system is preferred.

National triage scale

The British Association for Accident and Emergency Medicine and the A&E Nursing Association of the Royal College of Nursing have developed the national triage scale to be used in A&E Departments. A five point scale is used:

Colour	Priority	Category	Target time
Red	1	Immediate resuscitation	98% seen on arrival
Blue	2	Very urgent	95% seen within 10 min
Brown	3	Urgent	90% seen within 60 min
Yellow	4	Standard	Within 120 min
Green	5	Non-urgent	Within 240 min

Assignment to triage categories

1. The triage sieve. This is an initial triage tool for rapid categorization, usually of mass casualties

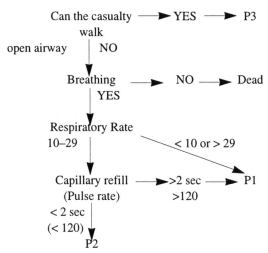

- The capillary refill time may be difficult to elicit due to environmental conditions.
- The triage sieve is not strictly applicable to children due to the physiological normal values used.
- The reliance on the patient's ability to walk may cause problems with the categorization of patients with isolated lower limb injuries.

2. *Triage revised trauma score (TRTS)* sometimes called the triage sort.

- The TRTS codes the three values, respiratory rate, systolic BP and the Glasgow Coma Scale as follows:

Respiratory rate	10–29	4
	> 29	3
	6–9	2
	1–5	1
	0	0
Systolic BP	> 90	4
	76–89	3
	50–75	2
	1–49	1
	0	0
Glasgow coma scale	13–15	4
	9–12	3
	6–8	2
	4–5	1
	3	0

The RTS is based on weighted values for the three parameters. The TRTS assigns a triage category based on the total unweighted score:

TRTS	Triage category
1–9	T1
10–11	T2
12	T3
0	T4

This method is simple and reproducible: the parameters and their scores are given on standard triage cards.

Triage labelling

Once a patient has been triaged, it is essential that he/she is labelled with the appropriate category. A wide range of labels are available of which the best is probably the Cambridge cruciform triage card. Other systems used are the BASICS card and the METAG card. If cards are not available, skin marking with indelible waterproof ink may be used.

Further reading

Advanced Life Support Group. *Major Incident Medical Management and Support.* London: BMJ Publishing, 1995.

Related topics of interest

UNITED KINGDOM TRAUMA OUTCOMES

There has been continuing debate on trauma management within the UK since the Royal College of Surgeons' report on the management of patients with major injuries in 1988. There remains little published evidence however, to suggest that trauma management has in fact objectively improved. A number of the report's recommendations have been introduced and studied in an attempt to measure change in trauma outcome relating to their implementation. These are principally the following.

National trauma audit

- The Major Trauma Outcome Study (now called the United Kingdom Trauma Audit and Research Network) began in 1988 and is co-ordinated by the North West Injuries Unit in Salford. (A similar scheme, The Scottish Trauma Audit Group was introduced in Scotland in 1992.)
- The project has been funded centrally by the Department of Health until the end of 1996. However, in the next 2 years allocation of funds will become the responsibility of the regional purchasers.
- There are now around 150 participating hospitals and approximately 50 000 patients on the national database.
- Entrance criteria are as follows:
  (a) Length of hospital stay greater than 72 h.
  (b) Hospital death.
  (c) Admission to an intensive care unit.

Patients with femoral neck and pubic rami fractures over 65 years and all isolated simple fractures are excluded.

- Analysis of the data uses the TRISS methodology (a logistic regression analysis of the injury severity score, RTS and the patient's age).
- Hospital and interhospital performance for trauma survival can be compared against a UK derived norm.

Trauma centres

- North Staffordshire Hospital was chosen to be a pilot trauma centre by the Department of Health in 1990. The aim was to evaluate the cost effectiveness and appropriateness of such a system within the UK.
- A 4-year study was undertaken by the Medical Care Research Unit at Sheffield University comparing North Staffordshire and surrounding region with hospitals with similar resources at Preston and Hull.
- The 4-year period spanned the introduction of the North Staffordshire trauma system.

- The aims of the study were to measure changes in processes of care, patient outcomes and cost effectiveness.
- The results of the comparative study published in 1996 showed no benefit in terms of cost, patient outcome and processes of care.

Helicopter transportation
- The London helicopter emergency medical service (HEMS) has been in operation since 1989.
- It has the capacity for two patients and is crewed by two pilots, a registrar grade doctor and a paramedic.
- It operates only in daylight hours and is activated by a paramedic at the London ambulance service control.
- The Medical Care Research Unit at Sheffield University assessed the impact of HEMS on trauma survival.
- A comparison was made during a 2-year period between patients who were attended to and transported by HEMS and a matched control group attended to by the London ambulance service paramedic crewed ambulances. The main outcome measure was survival at 6 months.
- There was no significant difference in survival between the two groups of patients in the study.

Further reading

Nicholl J, Turner J, Dixon S. *The Cost-Effectiveness of the Regional Trauma System in the North West Midlands. Medical Care Research Unit; Sheffield Centre for Health Related Research*. Sheffield: University of Sheffield, 1996.

Nicholl JP, Brazier JE, Snookes HA. Effects of London helicopter emergency medical services on survival after trauma. *British Medical Journal*, 1995; **311:** 217–22.

Yates DW, Woodford M, Hollis S. Preliminary analysis of the care of injured patients in 33 British hospitals: first report of the United Kingdom major trauma outcome study, *British Medical Journal*, 1992; **305:** 737–40.

Related topics of interest

Trauma scoring (p. 304)
Triage (p. 311)

VASCULAR TRAUMA

Traumatic vascular injury in the UK is uncommon. This is due to the low incidence of penetrating trauma in the UK (approximately 5% of all major trauma, compared to the USA where penetrating trauma accounts for approximately 40% of all major trauma).

Mechanism of injury

1. Iatrogenic. Principally from the increasing use of interventional radiography and cardiac catheterization, occasionally due to intra-arterial injection. This will not be considered further.

2. Penetrating trauma. Glass or stab wounds: such injuries are often associated with injuries to associated nerves and, in the extremities, tendons. Missile injuries: such injuries are usually associated with significant soft-tissue and bone injury due to cavitation and transfer of kinetic energy to surrounding tissues.

3. Blunt trauma. This can be direct, e.g. in association with a fracture, or indirect, e.g. secondary to a crushing or compression type of injury. As in the case of missile injuries, associated soft-tissue and bone injuries are common.

Assessment

Formal vascular assessment is a part of the secondary survey. Therefore attention should be paid to stabilizing the airway, breathing, circulation (including application of direct pressure to any bleeding points, but avoiding the use of tourniquets) and addressing any central neurological disability prior to proceeding to vascular assessment.

The clinical signs of vascular injury include:

- Pulsatile bleeding.
- Absent or reduced peripheral pulses.
- Distal ischaemia.
- Bruit.
- Expanding or pulsatile haematoma.

Other non-specific signs which should raise the suspicion of vascular injury include:

- Haematoma out of proportion to the local injury.
- Penetrating injury in the vicinity of a major vessel.
- Unexplained or disproportionate hypotension.
- Injury to a nerve or a tendon in the vicinity of a major vessel.

In addition, the patient may complain of one or more of the following:

- Pain: this may initially be attributed to local soft-tissue or bone injury.
- Numbness or coldness in an extremity: this may be attributed to peripheral nerve injury.

It is recognized that up to 25% of vascular injuries may be associated with palpable pulses on initial presentation. Repeated assessment of the patient with suspected vascular injury is therefore mandatory.

Patterns of injury

1. Open injury. Incomplete transection and puncture is caused by penetrating trauma or bone fragments in closed fractures. Presentation:

- Pulsatile haematoma.
- Delayed haemorrhage.

Sequelae (in cases of delayed diagnosis):

- False aneurysm.
- Rupture.
- Thrombosis.
- Embolism.
- Arterio-venous fistula.

Complete transection is usually secondary to penetrating trauma. Presentation:

- Haemorrhage.
- Haematoma.
- Distal ischaemia.
- Absent or reduced pulses.

Diagnosis is usually evident on initial clinical examination.

2. Closed injury. Usually due to a stretching injury from blunt trauma or to a compression injury (e.g. compression between the ends of bone fragments). Compartment syndrome may result from a closed injury to a relatively small vessel due to rising pressure from haemorrhage within a non-distensible compartment. Presentation:

- Distal ischaemia due to vessel occlusion (may be delayed, depending on mechanism of occlusion).

Occlusion may be caused by:

- Thrombosis: secondary to clot formation on exposed

intima secondary to an intimal tear, or from a subintimal dissection from a raised intimal flap leading to occlusion. Direct exploration is required to determine the cause of obstruction in such cases.

Investigations

1. Doppler ultrasound. A hand-held Doppler is sufficient to detect the presence of most traumatic vascular injuries. An absent signal indicates the need for immediate investigation, a reduced signal indicates that less urgency is present and treatment priorities may be established with other specialities, based upon the pattern and severity of other injuries.

2. Arteriography. Arteriography is used to:

- Exclude significant vascular injury.
- Define the site, nature and extent of vascular injury.
- Assess the patency of run-off vessels.

In the presence of clinical evidence of significant vascular injury, exploration should not be delayed in order to obtain an arteriogram.

Other indications for arteriography:

- Suspected partial tear of the aorta.
- Penetrating neck injuries.
- Displaced posterior fractures of the first rib.
- Clavicular injuries with signs of ischaemia.
- Recurrent bleed from the site of injury.
- A pulsatile mass or bruit suggestive of a false aneurysm or AV fistula.

Considerations in injuries to specific sites

1. Neck. Penetrating injuires to the neck with subsequent injury to the carotids may result in life-threatening compromise to the airway, breathing and circulation, due to expanding haematoma, haemopneumothorax or exsanguinating haematoma requiring immediate surgery. In the absence of such immediately life-threatening complications, arteriography is indicated prior to exploration.

2. Thoracic aorta. Rupture of the thoracic aorta should be suspected in all victims of blunt trauma where a significant deceleration force has been experienced (RTA or fall from a height). The most common radiological abnormality found in those reaching hospital alive is widening of the mediastinum. Liberal use of aortography in such cases will result in a diagnostic rate of approximately 10%.

3.   Intra-abdominal vessels. Control of massive intra-abdominal bleeding may be achieved by cross-clamping the supradiaphragmatic aorta via a left thoracotomy as a holding procedure while fluid resuscitation and preparation for urgent laparotomy are under way.

Further reading

Hocken DB. Acute vascular injury. *Surgery,* 1995; 44–8.
Welch GH. Vascular trauma. *Surgery,* 1990; 2068–73.

Related topics of interest

WHIPLASH INJURY

The term whiplash injury is used to describe the soft tissue injury resulting from a hyperextension (not hyperflexion) injury to the neck. The most common cause for such injuries is rear end shunts in road-traffic accidents, although collisions from other directions may cause identical injuries. Up to 42.6% of road-traffic accidents involve rear end shunts and an estimated 20% of occupants in such accidents will sustain some sort of neck injury.

Presenting symptoms

- Neck pain   98%.
- Occipital headache   72%.
- Shoulder pain   36%.
- Low back pain   35%.
- Interscapular pain   20%.
- Arm and hand pain   12%.
- Arm and hand numbness   12%.
- Vertigo   8%.
- Auditory   3%.
- Visual   1%.

20–25% of symptoms present late.

Severity of symptoms

Patients can be graded on a four point scale:

1. *Group A.* Asymptomatic.

2. *Group B.* Minor symptoms which do not interfere with work or leisure.

3. *Group C.* Symptoms which restrict leisure or work with or without frequent intermittent use of analgesia, orthotics or physiotherapy.

4. *Group D.* Loss of job, continuous use of analgesics, orthotics, repeated medical consultations. Other commonly reported symptoms include irritability, poor concentration and insomnia. Temperomandibular dysfunction may occur with pain, limitation of mouth opening and masticating muscle tenderness.

Clinical signs

Subjective neurological symptoms are common, definite neurological signs are less common. Horner's syndrome may occur rarely as a complication of whiplash injury.

Pattern of injury	The following injuries have been described in experimental animals subjected to hyperextension injuries and at post mortem in human victims of road traffic accidents:

- Muscle tears of sternomastoid and the paravertebral muscles.
- Retropharyngeal haematoma.
- Oesophageal contusion.
- Anterior longitudinal ligament tears.
- Cervical sympathetic chain injuries.
- Facet joint injury.
- Vertebral disc injury.

Investigations

Standard cervical spine views are usually normal. Flexion and extension views may show evidence of instability. MRI scanning may reveal significant soft tissue injury including ligamentous tears and disc herniation.

Prognosis

Approximately 46% of patients make a full recovery. Of the 44% who go on to have long-term symptoms approximately 10% are unable to work. The following factors are associated with poorer prognosis:

- Upper limb pain.
- Thoracolumbar pain.
- Increasing age.
- Presence of neurological signs.
- Pre-existing cervical spondylosis.
- Reversal of normal cervical lordosis on lateral c-spine film.
- Occipital headache.
- Female sex.
- Severity of initial pain.

The association between on-going litigation and the severity of symptoms and prognosis is controversial.

Long term prognosis

There have been several studies which have suggested that the incidence of cervical spondylosis is increased in those who have suffered a whiplash injury and that the age at onset of radiological changes of cervical spondylosis is less in those who have suffered a whiplash injury. However the methodology of such studies has been criticized and other studies have not confirmed these findings.

Treatment

Analgesia and early mobilization are the cornerstones of treatment of whiplash injuries. Studies suggest that early mobilization is at least as good as application of a cervical collar. Advice on mobilization exercises is as good as physiotherapy. The majority of patients will reach their final state of recovery within 2 months of injury, although some recovery in a proportionof patients may be expected for up to 1 year.

Further reading

Foy MA, Fagg PS. *Medicolegal Reporting in Orthopaedic Trauma.* Edinburgh: Churchill Livingstone, 1996.

Johnson, G. Hyperextension soft tissue injuries of the cervical spine – a review. *Journal of Accident and Emergency Medicine*, 1996; **13:** 3–8.

Related topics of interest

Brachial plexus injuries (p. 46)
Cervical spine injuries (p. 65)
Head injuries (p. 124)
Laryngeal fractures (p. 183)

WRIST FRACTURES

Fractures of the wrist account for approximately 20% of all new fracture-related out-patient attendances. Resulting most often from a fall on to an outstretched hand (FOOSH), they are most common in middle-aged and elderly females who suffer the predisposing factors of low bone density, unsteadiness and poor vision.

Colles fracture

Abraham Colles (1814) described a dorsally angulated fracture of the radius within 1 inch (2.5 cm) of the wrist joint.

Classification

The most commonly used method of classification is that described by Frykman in 1967, which is based on whether the fracture is intra- or extra-articular and whether it involves either or both of the distal radio-ulnar joint and the radio-carpal joint. This classification has been shown to be of value in predicting functional outcome.

Factors affecting stability include:

- Dorsal comminution.
- Dorsal angulation of 20° or more.
- Extensive intra-articular involvement.

Clinical features

The patient presents with a swollen, tender wrist which is painful to move. Bruising may occur. Classically there is a 'dinner fork' deformity due to dorsal angulation of the distal radius. However, this deformity may not be marked, or may be partially obscured by soft-tissue swelling. The possibility of scaphoid fracture, which is also classically caused by a fall on an outstretched hand, should not be overlooked.

In the case of displaced fractures, radiographs may demonstrate the following abnormalities:

- Impaction.
- Dorsal tilt.
- Radial displacement.
- Fracture of the ulnar styloid.
- Disruption of the inferior radio-ulnar joint.

Management: general considerations

The wrist plays an active role in hand movements, and therefore the principal aim of treatment of wrist fractures is to obtain optimal hand function on recovery. There is a direct relationship between residual deformity and poor hand function. The most important goal is to regain normal carpal alignment and, in particular, to avoid *dorsal* malalignment of the carpus.

Features influencing management decisions regarding methods of treatment include:

- Age of patient.
- Functional demand.
- General medical condition.
- Bone quality.
- Magnitude of soft-tissue injury.
- Fracture pattern.

All patients with wrist fractures should be given appropriate advice regarding initial rest and elevation followed by active finger, elbow and shoulder exercises.

Management: specific fracture patterns

1. Stable or undisplaced fractures. These fractures are managed in a plaster cast, usually a back slab in the first instance, with completion of plaster (or replacement by a synthetic cast) at 24 or 48 hours, at which time the soft-tissue swelling will be resolving. Immobilization is maintained for 5 weeks.

2. Displaced fractures. Displaced fractures which are stable after reduction are maintained in a below-elbow cast for 5 weeks. Stability is judged by the maintenance of a satisfactory closed reduction in plaster on post-reduction radiographs. Evidence of loss of position is an indication for further treatment, which will depend on the factors listed above.

3. Unstable fractures. Fractures which are unstable on initial closed manipulation are usually unstable following repeated such manipulations and attempts of this kind are best abandoned. K-wire stabilization may be used for extra-articular fractures or intra-articular fractures with one or two large fragments. This method can be supplemented by plaster or external fixation. Comminuted fractures are treated by external fixation between the radius proximal to the fracture and the second metacarpal shaft. The *Pennig* fixator has the advantage of allowing early wrist mobilization. In certain fractures, the external fixator can be joint sparing between the radius proximal to the fracture and the distal fragment proximal to the radio-carpal joint.

Complications

1. Early.

- Circulation: circulatory problems may occur as a result of a tight plaster.
- Damage to nerves: acute median nerve compression can occur and may require treatment by decompression.
- Reflex sympathetic dystrophy (Sudeck's atrophy): this is characterized by pain, stiffness and skin changes, including a shiny appearance, local tenderness and warmth. Later skin changes include coldness, sweating and blotchiness. Treatment includes intensive physiotherapy and guanethidine blocks. Referral to a pain clinic may be necessary.

2. Late.

- Malunion: occurs because of inadequate reduction or loss of position and produces a cosmetic abnormality along with loss of function and weakness. The commonest deformity is shortening of the radius, producing ulnar prominence, dorsal angulation and occasionally radial displacement. In selected cases excision of the lower end of the ulnar may improve function.
- Carpal tunnel syndrome.
- Rupture of extensor pollicis longus: usually seen after a few weeks in undisplaced or minimally displaced fractures. Treatment is by tendon transfer.
- Ulnar styloid tenderness: fibrous union of a fracture of the ulnar styloid may result in tenderness lasting weeks or very occasionally indefinately.
- Residual stiffness in neck and shoulder: these problems may follow a period of immobilization. Intensive physiotherapy may be helpful.

Smith's fracture

Robert Smith (1847) described an extra-articular fracture of the distal radius with volar (palmar) displacement. This fracture is sometimes known as a 'reversed Colles' and results from a fall on to a flexed wrist (for example when carrying shopping bags).

Clinical features

The clinical appearance may misleadingly resemble a dinner fork deformity, but careful examination will reveal the true nature of the displacement. The wrist is swollen, tender and bruised.

Treatment	Due to the inherent instability of these fractures, treatment is with open reduction and internal fixation with a volar T-buttress plate. Functional results are usually satisfactory.
Complications	These are similar to those seen in Colles fracture:

- Carpal tunnel syndrome.
- Malunion.
- Restricted function.
- Pain and stiffness.
- Reflex sympathetic dystrophy.

Barton's fracture

John Barton (1838) described a fracture of the distal radius through either the dorsal or volar aspect of the bone where the fracture involves the joint line. These fractures, particularly when displaced, need fixation to restore congruity of the joint line. The complications are as for Smith's fracture.

Scaphoid fracture

These are common injuries, usually resulting from a fall on to an outstretched hand. They tend to be rare in children (who suffer epiphyseal injuries) and in the elderly (who are more likely to suffer a Colles fracture).

Scaphoid injuries are easily overlooked, with potentially serious consequences. The blood supply to the scaphoid enters the bone distally resulting in a poor proximal supply. As a consequence of this, the bone is at risk of avascular necrosis of the proximal part with fractures of the waist of the scaphoid.

Clinical features	
	• Tenderness in the anatomical snuffbox (alone, this is relatively non-specific).
	• Pain on longitudinal pressure along the thumb (axial compression).
	• Tenderness over the dorsum of the scaphoid.
	• Pain on wrist movement.

Radiological appearances	Specific scaphoid views must be requested. Initial films may be normal, in which case repeat films at 10–14 days may reveal a fracture.
Management	The most common fractures are of the waist of the scaphoid and are managed in a 'scaphoid' plaster for 6 weeks. Displaced fractures are uncommon and require open fixation with a Herbert screw.

When the initial radiographs are normal and a fracture is suspected, the wrist is immobilized in a double tubigrip, Futura® splint or plaster, depending on the degree of pain. Radiography is repeated at 10 or 14 days. If the repeat films confirm a fracture, it is immobilized in plaster (or a synthetic cast) for 6 weeks. If the repeat film is normal, but scaphoid tenderness persists, a nuclear bone scan should be performed to confirm or exclude fracture. If this is not done, the patient is likely to be subjected to long periods of unnecessary immobilization and repeated radiography or risk a missed fracture.

A syndrome of persisting pain despite negative investigations, which fails to respond to any treatment, occurs in young women.

Complications

- Delayed union: treated by bone grafting and screw fixation.
- Non-union: treated by bone grafting and screw fixation.
- Avascular necrosis: this is due to compromised blood supply (see above). The proximal fragment appears dense on radiography. Surgery may involve excision of the dense fragment or selected carpal fusion.
- Osteo-arthritis: usually occurs due to avascular necrosis. Arthrodesis may be necessary.

Carpal dislocation

The most common injury patterns are:

- Lunate and perilunate dislocation.
- Scapho-lunate dislocation.

These patterns are diagnosed by careful interpretation of radiographs, paying particular attention to whether the lunate is correctly sited between the radius and the remainder of the carpus. If such an injury is suspected, expert orthopaedic assistance is required, and the dislocation should be reduced and the reduction maintained for at least 4 weeks.

Wrist injuries in children

The wrist is the most common site for greenstick fractures in children, resulting from the same mechanism as Colles fracture in adults (fall on an outstretched hand).

- Displaced fractures require closed reduction and plaster of Paris immobilization.
- Epiphyseal injuries are also common at the wrist, commonly Salter-Harris types 1 and 2 (*Figure 1*).

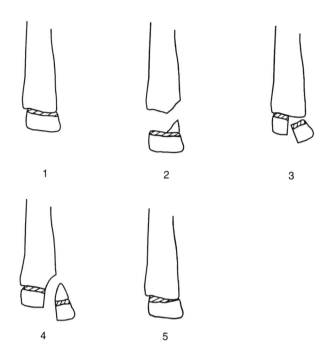

Figure 1. Salter-Harris classification of epiphyseal plate injuries. Type 1, the whole epiphysis is separated from the shaft. Type 2, the epiphysis is displaced, carrying with it a small, triangular metaphyseal fragment (the most common injury). Type 3, separation of part of the epiphysis. Type 4, separation of part of the epiphysis, with a metaphyseal fragment. Type 5, crushing of part of the epiphysis. Adapted from Burke, Greaves and Hormbrey (1995) *Self Assessment in Accident and Emergency Medicine,* Butterworth Heinemann.

- Complete fractures of the distal radius and ulnar in children are often difficult to reduce and occasionally K-wire stabilization is necessary.
- The most common complication is malunion, the majority of cases of which will resolve spontaneously with growth and remodelling.

Further reading

Dandy DJ. *Essential Orthopaedics and Trauma,* 2nd Edn. Edinburgh: Churchill Livingstone, 1993.

Related topics of interest

INDEX

ORDERING DETAILS

Main address for orders

BIOS Scientific Publishers Ltd
9 Newtec Place, Magdalen Road,
Oxford OX4 1RE, UK
Tel: +44 1865 726286
Fax: +44 1865 246823

Australia and New Zealand
Blackwell Science Asia
54 University Street, Carlton, South Victoria 3053, Australia
Tel: (3) 9347 0300
Fax: (3) 9347 5001

India
Viva Books Private Ltd
4325/3 Ansari Road, Daryaganj, New Delhi 110 002, India
Tel: 11 3283121
Fax: 11 3267224

Singapore and South East Asia
(Brunei, Hong Kong, Indonesia, Korea, Malaysia, the Philippines,
Singapore, Taiwan, and Thailand)
Toppan Company (S) PTE Ltd
38 Liu Fang Road, Jurong, Singapore 2262
Tel: (265) 6666
Fax: (261) 7875

USA and Canada
BIOS Scientific Publishers
PO Box 605, Herndon, VA 20172-0605, USA
Tel: (703) 661 1500
Fax: (703) 661 1501

Payment can be made by cheque or credit card (Visa/Mastercard, quoting number
and expiry date). Alternatively, a *pro forma* invoice can be sent.

Prepaid orders must include £2.50/US$5.00 to cover postage and packing
(two or more books sent post free)